Peter V. Giannoudis

Editor

Practical Procedures in Elective Orthopaedic Surgery

Upper Extremity and Spine

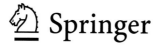 Springer

Editor
Peter V. Giannoudis, B.Sc., M.B., M.D., FRCS
Academic Department of Trauma
and Orthopaedic Surgery
School of Medicine
University of Leeds
Leeds
UK

ISBN 978-0-85729-819-5   e-ISBN 978-0-85729-820-1
DOI 10.1007/978-0-85729-820-1
Springer London Dordrecht Heidelberg New York

British Library Cataloguing in Publication Data
A catalogue record for this book is available from the British Library

Library of Congress Control Number: 2011941598

Printed on acid-free paper

Springer is part of Springer Science+Business Media (www.springer.com)

Practical Procedures in Elective Orthopaedic Surgery

To my wife Rania, my children Marilena and Vasilis
Whom
I have missed so much during my medical career.
I thank them for providing me with ongoing inspiration and support.
Their love has been a source of endless energy and creativity.

Preface

A plethora of Orthopaedic Textbooks have been produced over the years presenting the advances made in this ever evolving discipline. Some of them being colossal cover the entire practice of orthopaedic surgery, whereas others include only regional orthopaedics by focusing into a specific anatomical site of the musculoskeletal system.

The idea of the book was conceived during the beginning of my residency program in orthopaedic surgery. Moving every 6 months to a different subspecialty, it became clear that I had to obtain different textbooks in order to use them as a quick, yet comprehensive reference, prior to performing a surgical procedure.

Following the development and the popularity of the trauma textbook, I felt obliged to also develop a similar book in elective orthopaedic surgery that would contain a stepwise approach related to these types of surgical procedures. In this textbook, the most common procedures that a surgeon in training is expected to perform during his residency program for the upper extremity and the spine have been included. Each procedure has been written by an expert or under a supervision of an expert. Each chapter provides such useful information to the trainee as indications, clinical and radiological assessment, surgical approach, implant positioning, tips and tricks, postoperative complications to be aware of, mode of mobilisation and the time intervals of outpatient follow up. Intra-operative pictures have been incorporated to allow the surgeon to be aware of all the important issues and steps involved for each procedure.

This book by no means covers all the procedures to be performed during a residency program. The objective was not to become cumbersome, but rather the textbook to be easy to carry and simple to read. It is expected to be the companion for the resident in training and to improve the standard of care of our patients that we care so much about.

Leeds, UK   Peter V. Giannoudis B.Sc., M.B., M.D., FRCS

Acknowledgments

Without the dedication and the hard work of my Hospital Staff and my colleagues it would not have been possible to complete this project.

I would also personally like to thank all the contributors who have shared with me their expertise.

Contents

Contributors

Arup K. Bhadra, M.D. Academic Department of Trauma and Orthopaedics, School of Medicine, University of Louisville, Louisville, KY, USA

Frank O. Bonnarens, M.D. Academic Department of Trauma and Orthopaedics, School of Medicine, University of Louisville, Louisville, KY, USA

Grainne Bourke, FRCSI, FRCS (Plast) Department of Plastic and Reconstructive Surgery, Leeds Teaching Hospitals NHS Trust, Leeds, UK

Doug A. Campbell, ChM, FRCS-Ed (Orth), FFSEM (UK) Department of Trauma and Orthopaedic Surgery, Leeds Teaching Hospitals NHS Trust, Leeds, UK

Robert A. Dunsmuir, B.Sc. (Hons), MBChB, FRCS-Ed (Orth) Department of Trauma and Orthopaedic Surgery, Leeds Teaching Hospitals NHS Trust, Leeds, UK

Robert Farnell, M.B.B.S., FRCS-Eng, FRCS (Orth) Department of Trauma and Orthopaedic Surgery, Leeds Teaching Hospitals NHS Trust, Leeds, UK

Peter V. Giannoudis, B.Sc., M.D., FRCS-Eng Academic Department of Trauma and Orthopaedic Surgery, School of Medicine, University of Leeds, Leeds, UK

Roger Hackney, FRCS (Orth) Department of Trauma and Orthopaedic Surgery, Leeds Teaching Hospitals NHS Trust, Leeds, UK

Nikolaos K. Kanakaris, M.D., Ph.D. Department of Trauma and Orthopaedic Surgery, Leeds Teaching Hospitals NHS Trust, Leeds, UK

Efthimios J. Karadimas, M.D., Ph.D. Department of Trauma and Orthopaedic Surgery, Leeds Teaching Hospitals NHS Trust, Leeds, UK

George M. Kontakis, M.D., Ph.D. Academic Department of Trauma and Orthopaedic Surgery, School of Medicine, University of Crete, Heraclion, Crete, Greece

Panagiotis Liantis, M.D., Third Academic Department of Trauma and Orthopaedic Surgery, School of Medicine, University of Athens, Athens, Greece

David Limb, B.Sc., FRCS-Ed (Orth) Leeds General Infirmary, Leeds, UK

Antony L.R. Michael, DNB (T&O), M.Sc., FRCS (Orth) Department of Trauma and Orthopaedics, Leeds Teaching Hospitals NHS Trust, Leeds, UK

Abhay S. Rao, FRCS (Orth) Department of Spinal Surgery, Leeds Teaching Hospitals NHS Trust, Leeds, UK

Craig S. Roberts, M.D., FACS Academic Department of Trauma and Orthopaedics, School of Medicine, University of Louisville, Louisville, KY, USA

Emilio Delli Sante, M.D. Department of Trauma and Orthopaedic Surgery, Leeds Teaching Hospitals NHS Trust, Leeds, UK

Christos Sinopidis, M.D. 'St. Luke's' Hospital, Thessaloniki, Greece

Panayotis N. Soucacos, M.D., FACS Academic Department of Trauma and Orthopaedic Surgery, School of Medicine, University of Athens, Athens, Greece

Panagiotis Stavlas, M.D. Department of Trauma and Orthopaedics, 'Thriassio' General Hospital, Elefsina, Greece

Jake Timothy, M.D. Department of Neurosurgery, Leeds Teaching Hospitals NHS Trust, Leeds, UK

Theodoros I. Tosounidis, M.D., EEC (Orth) Department of Trauma and Orthopaedic Surgery, Leeds Teaching Hospitals NHS Trust, Leeds, UK

Andrew Williams, M.B.B.S. Department of Plastic and Reconstructive Surgery, Leeds Teaching Hospitals NHS Trust, Leeds, UK

Fragkiskos N. Xypnitos, M.D., M.Sc., Ph.D., EEC (Orth) Department of Trauma and Orthopaedics, Leeds Teaching Hospitals NHS Trust, Leeds, UK

Part I

Upper Extremity: Clavicle – Shoulder

Treatment of Nonunion of Clavicle Fractures

1

Peter V. Giannoudis, Emilio Delli Sante, and Fragkiskos N. Xypnitos

Indications

- Painful nonunion following non-operative treatment.
- Painful nonunion following open reduction and internal fixation.

Preoperative Planning

Clinical Assessment

- Assess local deformity and state of soft tissues.
- Define clearly previous incision(s), and plan new incision.
- Assess and document vascular status of the upper extremity and any difference in peripheral pulses between the nonunion and contralateral extremity.

P.V. Giannoudis (✉)
Academic Department of Trauma and Orthopaedic Surgery,
School of Medicine, University of Leeds,
Leeds, UK
e-mail: pgiannoudi@aol.com

E.D. Sante
Department of Trauma and Orthopaedic Surgery,
Leeds Teaching Hospitals NHS Trust,
Leeds, UK

F.N. Xypnitos
Department of Trauma and Orthopaedics,
Leeds Teaching Hospitals NHS Trust,
Leeds, UK

- Assess the neurological status of the upper extremity (usually previous brachial plexus injury presents as an upper roots traction injury).

Radiological Assessment

- Anteroposterior view of the clavicle including the sternoclavicular and acromioclavicular joints (Fig. 1.1).
- Oblique views.
- Assess state of metal work form previous ORIF procedure.

Operative Treatment

Anesthesia

- General anesthesia.
- Administration of prophylactic antibiotics as per local hospital protocol at induction.
- If there is concern about the presence of low grade infection, do not administer antibiotics until obtaining intra-operative cultures.

Table and Equipment

- AO small fragment (3.5 mm) set.
- Ensure availability of the pre-planned plate length. A 3.5 DCP plate or a reconstruction plate can be used (Fig. 1.2a, b).
- Standard osteosynthesis set as per local hospital protocol.

P.V. Giannoudis (ed.), *Practical Procedures in Elective Orthopaedic Surgery*,
DOI 10.1007/978-0-85729-820-1_1, © Springer-Verlag London Limited 2012

Fig. 1.1 A clavicular nonunion due to hardware failure

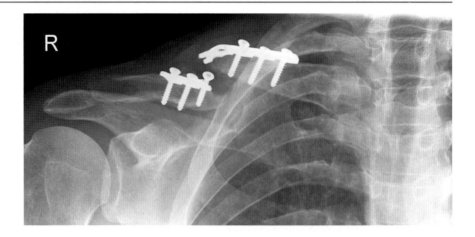

Table Set up

- The instrumentation is set-up on the side of the operation.
- Image intensifier is from the ipsilateral side.
- Position the table diagonally across the operating room so that the operating area lies in the clean air field.

Draping and Surgical Approach

- Beach-chair positioning of the patient (Fig. 1.3).
- Skin preparation is carried out using usual antiseptic solutions (aqueous/alcoholic povidone-iodine).
- Prepare the skin of the chest to the medial border of the scapula. Clean up to the anterior and lateral surface of the neck and down below the level of the nipple.
- Use single U-drapes.
- Make an incision over the clavicle or use previous incision (Fig. 1.4a, b).
- Using the cutting diathermy, expose the broken plate or the nonunion site (Fig. 1.5a).
- Remove the metal work (Fig. 1.5b), and debride the fibrous tissue at the nonunion site.
- Prepare a healthy (bleeding) soft tissue and bone bed.
- Drill the IM canal of both segments of the nonunion with a 2.5-cm drill (Fig. 1.6).
- Drill a hole to the bone through a plate hole above the distal fragment, and fix the plate to the distal fragment.

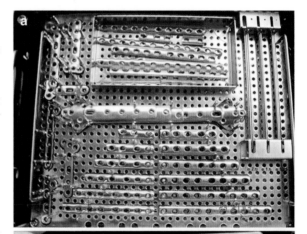

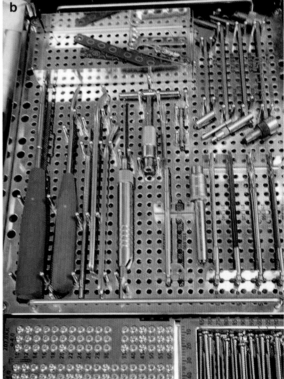

Fig. 1.2 (**a** and **b**) A 3.5 DCP or a reconstruction plating system can be used

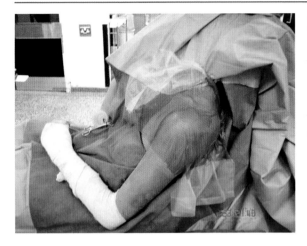

Fig. 1.3 The position of the table is the beach chair, taking in consideration the possible necessity of X-rays through the operation

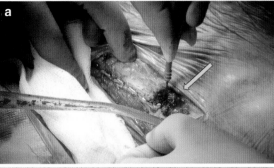

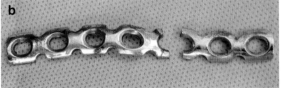

Fig. 1.5 (**a**) Exposure of the broken plate, the *arrow* points the nonunion site. (**b**) The removed broken plate

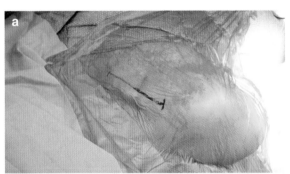

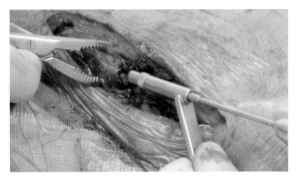

Fig. 1.6 Using a 2.5mm drill the medullary canal of the clavicle can be opened allowing the subsequent mobilisation of osteo-progenitor cells at the site of the non-union

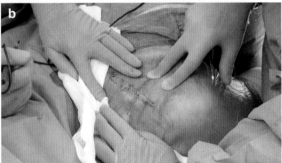

Fig. 1.4 (**a**) Skin marking and (**b**) incision

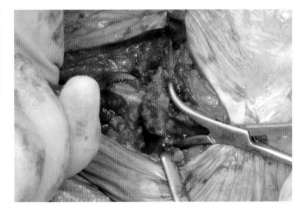

Fig. 1.7 Reduction of the nonunion prior of plate positioning

- Then reduce the proximal fragment (Fig. 1.7), and secure the plate positioning over the bone by using a clamp.
- Insert one screw at the proximal fragment, and ensure reduction is maintained.
- Insert the remaining screws.
- Cancellous bone grafting is performed for bone defects or devitalized bone (Fig. 1.8a, b).
- Ensure fracture reduction and appropriate screw length with fluoroscopic lordotic views.

Closure

- Closure is performed as a full-thickness layer over the plate using 2/0 Vicryl and 3/0 subcuticular sutures for the skin (Fig. 1.9a, b).

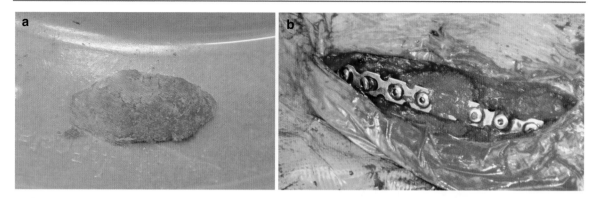

Fig. 1.8 (**a**) Cancellous bone graft + BMP used in this case. (**b**) The graft is placed at the nonunion site

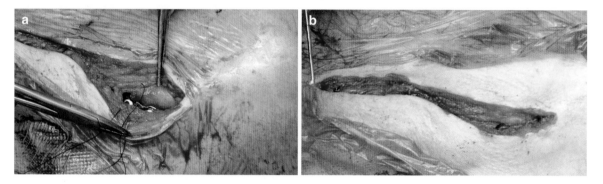

Fig. 1.9 (**a**) Wound closure with continuous suturing technique (**b**) covering the plate

Fig. 1.10 Post operative X-ray of the clavicular non-union stabilised with a reconstruction plate

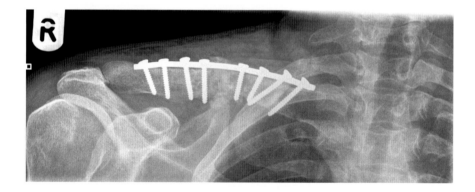

Postoperative Treatment

- Assess and document the neurovascular status of the upper extremity.
- Obtain postoperative radiographs (Fig. 1.10).
- Use a sling for the first 10 postoperative days (Fig. 1.11).
- Initiate active flexion and abduction 4–6 weeks after injury.
- Return to prior activities within 12 weeks from the time of surgery when clinical and radiological union has been confirmed.

Outpatient Follow-up

- Review at clinic at 6, 12 weeks, and at 6 months with X-rays on arrival.
- Beware of late vascular complications (thrombosis; pseudoaneurysm).

Implant Removal

- Plate can be removed following osseous union after a minimum period of 9 months.

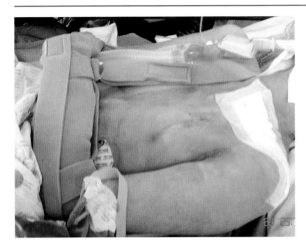

Fig. 1.11 The sling, used for the first 10 post-op days

Further Reading

Khan SA, Shamshery P, Gupta V, et al. Locking compression plate in long standing clavicular nonunions with poor bone stock. J Trauma. 2008;64(2):439–41.

Kirmani SJ, Pillai SK, Madegowda BR, et al. Vertical fragment in adult midshaft clavicle fractures: an indicator for surgical intervention. Orthopedics. 2009;32(10):pii.

Kloen P, Werner CM, Stufkens SA, et al. Anteroinferior plating of midshaft clavicle nonunions and fractures. Oper Orthop Traumatol. 2009;21(2):170.

Rosenberg N, Neumann L, Wallace AW. Functional outcome of surgical treatment of symptomatic nonunion and malunion of midshaft clavicle fractures. J Shoulder Elbow Surg. 2007;16(5):510–3.

McKee MD, Wild LM, Schemitsch EH. Midshaft malunions of the clavicle. Surgical technique. J Bone Joint Surg Am. 2004;86-A Suppl 1:37–43.

Acromioclavicular Joint Dislocation

2

Roger Hackney, Fragkiskos N. Xypnitos, and Peter V. Giannoudis

Indications

- Rockwood and Tossy classification grades 4–6. Type 3 does no better with surgery than with conservative treatment.
- Chronic pain after at least 9 months of conservative treatment.
- In my experience, many failures of conservative treatment were not type 3.

Preoperative Planning

Clinical Assessment

- History of discomfort and reduced shoulder function, grating and grinding plus dissatisfaction with the cosmetic appearance.

R. Hackney (✉)
Department of Trauma and Orthopaedic Surgery,
Leeds Teaching Hospitals NHS Trust,
Leeds, UK
e-mail: roger.hackne@leedsth.nhs.uk

F.N. Xypnitos
Department of Trauma and Orthopaedics,
Leeds Teaching Hospitals NHS Trust,
Leeds, UK

P.V. Giannoudis
Academic Department of Trauma and Orthopaedic Surgery,
School of Medicine,University of Leeds,
Leeds, UK

- Examination shows a displaced lateral end of clavicle that may or may not be reducible.

Radiological Assessment

- Plain AP radiographs will demonstrate the degree of vertical displacement and any coexisting fracture (Fig. 2.1).
- Calcification of the coracoacromio ligament will be demonstrated.
- Plain AP films do not give an idea of the degree of posterior displacement that often gives rise to an unsatisfactory result from conservative treatment.
- I do not use the classic weight-bearing film, preferring clinical examination.

Operative Treatment

Anesthesia

- General anesthesia with interscalene block.
- Hypotensive anesthesia.

Table and Equipment

- Basic instruments, plus retractor, osteotomes, drill, saw, specific instrumentation for artificial implant, and AO small fragment set.

P.V. Giannoudis (ed.), *Practical Procedures in Elective Orthopaedic Surgery*,
DOI 10.1007/978-0-85729-820-1_2, © Springer-Verlag London Limited 2012

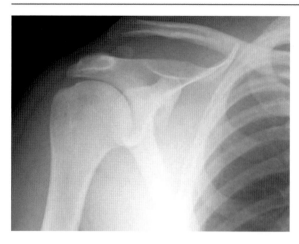

Fig. 2.1 AP radiograph demonstrating the degree of vertical displacement and a co-existing fracture

Table Set up

- Instruments the same side as the surgeon within the clean air environment.

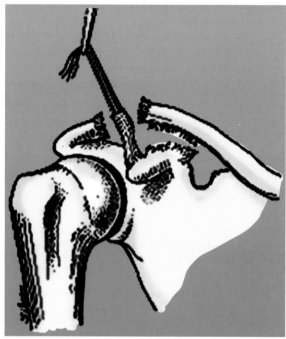

Fig. 2.2 The coracoacromial ligament is harvested on a 0.5 cm cubed piece of acromion, which is then held with a 5 ethibond suture

Patient Positioning

- Shoulder table with positioner, e.g., Mayfield head ring or Schlein support.
- Patient is semi-reclined with the arm by the side.

Draping and Surgical Approach

- Prepare the skin and use a U-drape to shut off the operative field.
- An iodine-soaked swab is left in the axilla. A Ioban is used.
- A sabre or bra-strap incision is made 1–2 cm medial to the lateral end of the clavicle, extending halfway to the coracoid.
- Skin flaps are raised above the clavipectoral fascia.
- A T incision is made on the clavicle, based on the lateral end, with subperiosteal elevation of muscle, fascia, and capsule.
- The remaining capsule/scar attached to the clavicle is dissected free.

- Using two Trethowan retractors to protect underlying tissues, the lateral 1–2 cm of the lateral ends of the clavicle are removed with a saw.
- The coracoacromial ligament is palpated under the deltoid and dissected free to the edge of the acromion.
- A small osteotome is used to harvest the ligament on a 0.5 cm cubed piece of acromion, which is then held with a 5 ethibond suture (Fig. 2.2).
- A number of devices are commercially available to provide reconstruction of the coracoacromial ligaments. Become familiar with one.
- The coracoid is then approached by the deltopectoral groove, preserving the cephalic vein.
- A pair of curved clips, such as Lahey's, is then used to define a passage between the conjoined tendon and pectoralis minor, allowing the insertion of a finger, palpating the undersurface of the coracoid.
- The guide drill for the device can then be passed safely through clavicle then into or around the coracoid.

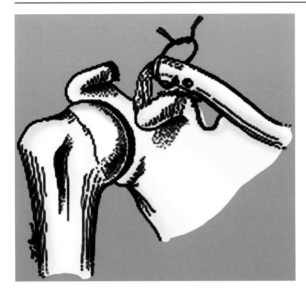

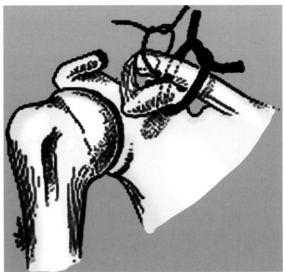

Fig. 2.3 The 5 ethibond suture is passed through the hole in the superior cortex of the clavicle and the bone on the end of the coracoacromial ligament secured into the cavity in the clavicle as the suture is tied

Fig. 2.4 A suture fixation can be used for additional support to the repair

- The device is tightened and the clavicle reduced.
- A pair of nibblers is used to excavate a cavity in the medulla of the clavicle. A small drill or bone awl is used to make a hole in the superior cortex of the clavicle. The needle of the 5 ethibond suture is passed through this, and the bone on the end of the coracoacromial ligament is secured into the cavity in the clavicle as the suture is tied (Fig. 2.3).
- An additional partially threaded cancellous screw, a Bosworth type screw, with a washer or a suture fixation (Fig. 2.4) can then be used for additional support to the repair. This is used for patients who may not comply with the postoperative instructions, but does require a second operation for removal of screw at 6 weeks.
- The capsule of the reconstructed joint and the clavi-pectoral fascia are closed with 1 ethibond. Fat is closed with Vicryl.
- A subcuticular stitch is used for skin.

Postoperative Rehabilitation

- A sling is worn for up to 6 weeks depending upon the reliability of the patient.
- No heavy lifting, pushing or overhead activity is permitted for 6 weeks.

Follow-up

- It is advisable that the patient will be followed for the next, 2, 4 weeks, and the following 3 and 6 months prior to discharge.

Further Reading

Lafosse L, Baier GP, Leuzinger J. Arthroscopic treatment of acute and chronic acromioclavicular joint dislocation. Arthroscopy. 2005;21(8):1017.

Ogilvie-Harris DJ, D'Angelo G. Arthroscopic surgery of the shoulder. Sports Med. 1990;9(2):120–8.

Diagnostic Shoulder Arthroscopy

3

Roger Hackney

Indications

- Stabilization procedures; labral repair, capsular placation, SLAP repairs, closure of rotator interval, and posterior stabilization.
- Rotator cuff disease; impingement, rotator cuff repair, removal of calcific deposits.
- Acromioplasty.
- Excision lateral end of clavicle.
- Debridement, synovectomy.
- Treatment of cartilage defects.
- Removal of loose bodies.
- Capsular release for adhesive capsulitis/shoulder stiffness.
- Remove tip of coracoid for subcoracoid impingement.

Preoperative Planning

Clinical Assessment

- Typical shoulder complaints include:
  - Sensations of instability.
  - Painful loss of range of motion affecting ability to dress/undress, manage hair, driving.
  - Night pain.
  - Weakness.

- Loss of internal and external rotation and overhead activity.

Radiological Assessment

- Plain film in two planes, typically an anteroposterior view and axillary view. Other specialized views may be required for some conditions (Fig. 3.1).
- Ultrasound scan; a dynamic investigation that provides information principally for rotator cuff disease and subacromial impingement.
- MRI scan with arthrogram. Frequently used for investigation of instability, but surgeons should proceed to arthroscopy on clinical grounds.
- CT scan; used to investigate size of bony defects in instability work-up.

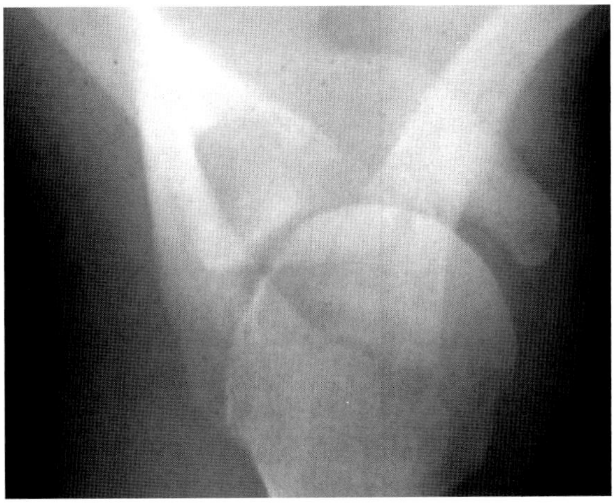

Fig. 3.1 Axillary view revealing loss of anterior glenoid in a recurrent dislocation

R. Hackney
Department of Trauma and Orthopaedic Surgery,
Leeds Teaching Hospitals NHS Trust,
Leeds, UK
e-mail: roger.hackney@leedsth.nhs.uk

P.V. Giannoudis (ed.), *Practical Procedures in Elective Orthopaedic Surgery*,
DOI 10.1007/978-0-85729-820-1_3, © Springer-Verlag London Limited 2012

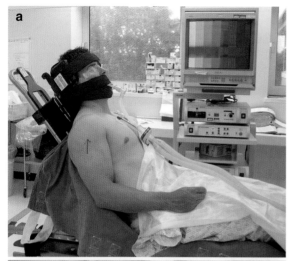

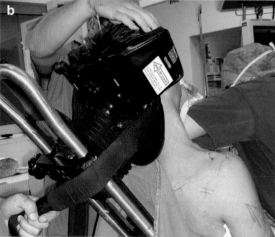

Fig. 3.2 (a) Beach chair position. (b) Head ring support

Operative Treatment

Anesthesia

- Regional (interscalene block) and/or general anesthesia.
- Hypotensive, systolic blood pressure below 100 mmHg.
- Antibiotic prophylaxis required if implants used.

Patient Positioning

- Debate as to which position is better.
- Beach chair (Fig. 3.2a):
  - Use of Head ring or table support such as Schlein (Fig. 3.2b).

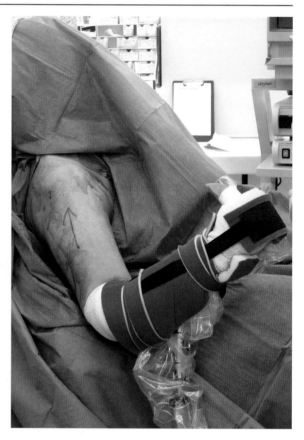

Fig. 3.3 Traction device

- Advantages of beach chair:
  Shoulder is in upright position, therefore position of instruments and anatomy is more intuitive for operative procedures.
  Easier conversion to open procedures.
  Short set-up time.
  Requires use of an assistant or traction device (Fig. 3.3) to apply traction.
- Lateral position:
  - Lateral supports, traction equipment fixed to table.
  - Advantages of lateral position:
  Greater traction can be applied in more than one plane.

Arthroscopy Equipment

- Arthroscope with high flow cannula
- Camera stack system with light source, high definition television screen, photograph/video recording system for images (Fig. 3.4a).
- Arthroscopic pump and shaver (Fig. 3.4b).

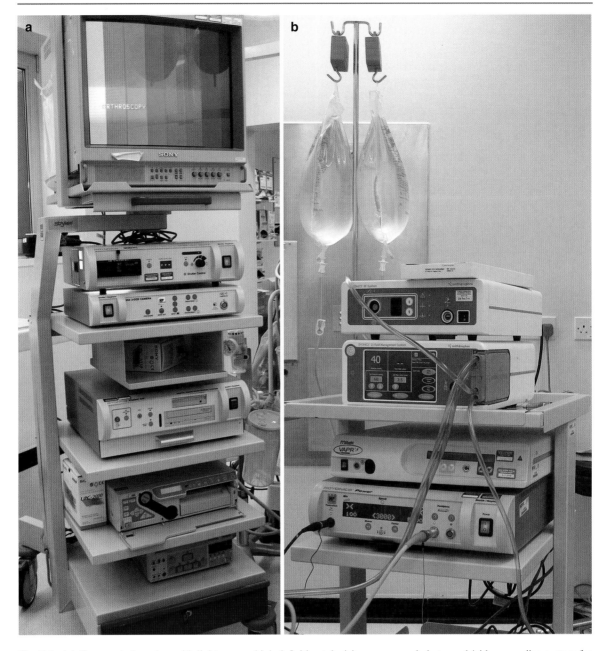

Fig. 3.4 (**a**) Camera stack system with light source, high definition television screen, and photograph/video recording system for images. (**b**) Arthroscopic pump and shaver

- Electrocautery.
- Arthroscopic instruments (Fig. 3.5a–c).

Set-up

- Camera at the opposite side of the table.
- Arthroscopic instruments at the same side of the table.

Draping and Surgical Approach

- Mark the anatomy preoperatively, including the spine of the scapula, acromion process, coracoid, humeral head, and clavicle. Mark the typical arthroscopy portals (Fig. 3.6).
- An examination under anesthesia (EUA) should be performed comparing both shoulders for range of

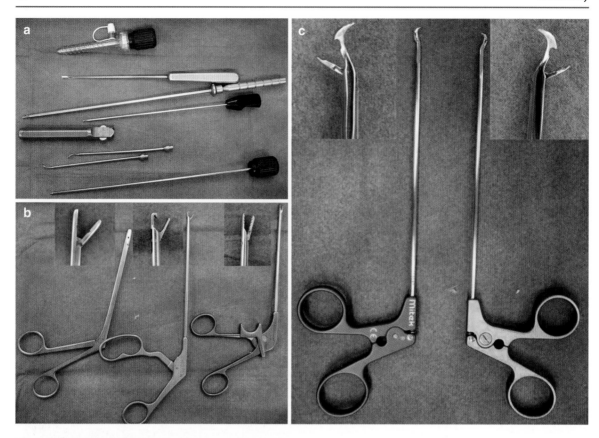

Fig. 3.5 (**a–c**) Arthroscopic instruments

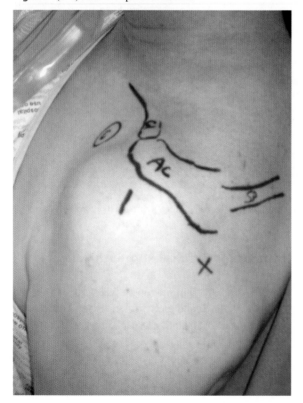

Fig. 3.6 Marked portals

motion and joint laxity in three planes, anterior, inferior, and posterior.

- Skin preparation with antiseptic solution (Fig. 3.7).
- U-drape allowing exposure of the whole of the shoulder joint and arm.
- The standard entry point for the arthroscope is 2.5 cm inferior and medial to the posterolateral corner of the acromion, in the soft spot between infra and supraspinatus.
- The initial incision is with a no. 11 blade pointing toward the coracoid process (Fig. 3.8).
- The arthroscopic trocar is introduced pointing toward the coracoid process of the scapula (Fig. 3.9a).
- Holding the trocar in one hand, the other hand is used to grip and manipulate the humeral head. The trocar can then be felt to move against the humeral head, slide along infraspinatus to the "soft spot." Too medial, and the trocar presses against the back of the neck of the glenoid, this is palpably more solid than the head of the humerus which can be balloted by the free hand.
- Once the soft spot is confirmed, firm pressure on the trocar towards the coracoid will lead to a sudden give as the trocar enters the glenohumeral joint.

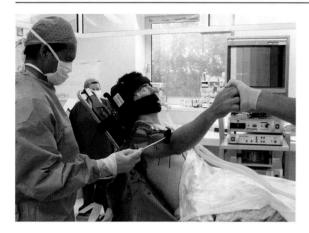

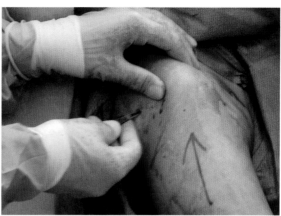

Fig. 3.7 Skin preparation

Fig. 3.8 The initial incision with a no. 11 blade pointing toward the coracoid process

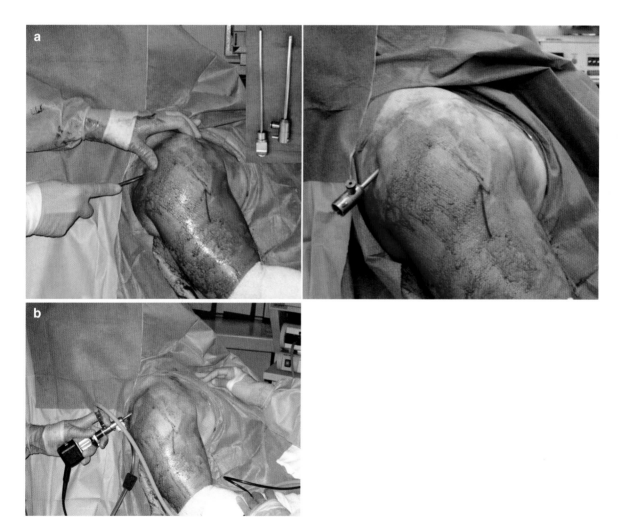

Fig. 3.9 (**a**) Insertion of the arthroscopic trocar pointing towards the coracoid process of the scapula. (**b**) Introduction of the arthroscope

Fig. 3.10 (**a**) Supraspinatus (*SS*), humeral head (*H*) and long head of biceps (*LHB*). (**b**) A Hill Sachs lesion (*HSL*). (**c**) A type I SLAP lesion (*arrow*). (**d**) Labral degenerative tear (*L* labrum, *IGHL* inferior gleno-humeral ligament)

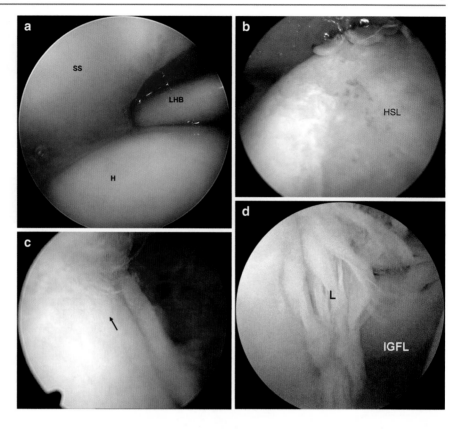

There is great variability in the resistance, and hence force required between individuals. The arthroscope is introduced into the trocar, and the fluid line opened (Fig. 3.9b). The theater lights should be dimmed.

Inspection of the Glenohumeral Joint

- A routine for joint inspection is undertaken. The technique recommended by ISAKOS is advised.
  - The long head of biceps (LHB) is identified and followed out to the rotator cuff (Fig. 3.10a).
  - The insertion of subscapularis, supraspinatus, and infraspinatus are inspected.
  - The sling holding the long head of biceps, and superior glenohumeral ligament are noted.
  - Posteriorly, the site of the impaction fracture of anterior dislocation (Hill-Sachs lesion) is observed (Fig. 3.10b).
  - The LHB is traced back to its origin on the superior glenoid labrum and any SLAP lesion found (Fig. 3.10c).

- At this stage, it may be necessary to introduce a probe into the joint. The arthroscope is moved anteriorly to a preferred site of entry for the probe. The light from the arthroscope is seen through the anterior shoulder, and an incision made at that point. The probe is then introduced by direct observation with the arthroscope. The probe can be used to assess the freedom of the LHB, the integrity of its attachment to the glenoid and the continuity of the glenoid labrum.
  - The arthroscope is moved inferiorly from the superior labrum to inspect the rotator interval and middle glenohumeral ligament (if present), then trace the anterior labrum to the origin of the inferior glenohumeral ligament and the inferior labrum (Fig. 3.10d).
  - The inferior recess can be inspected either from an anterior position in the presence of a lax shoulder, or by following the posterior labrum down from the LHB attachment into the recess. A formal inspection of the joint surfaces should be made.

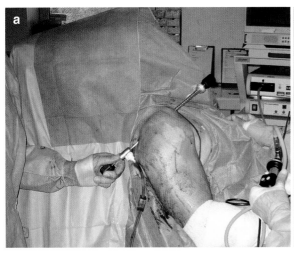
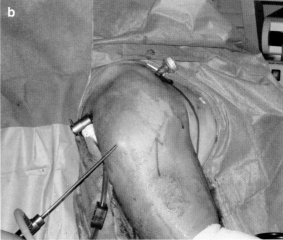

Fig. 3.11 (**a**, **b**) "Switching stick" technique

Bursoscopy

- The arthroscope is removed from the cannula, and the trocar re-inserted.
- The trocar is removed from the joint as far as the surface of the rotator cuff.
- The angle of insertion is then towards the posterior surface of the acromion.
- The trocar is slid over the cuff into the subacromial space.
- Moving the trocar from side to side will confirm the position under the acromion.
- The arthroscope is inserted into the cannula, and the fluid switched on.
- The arthroscope is frequently not within the bursa, but above or below. The bursa is a free space without the flimsy film of tissue seen outside the bursa.
- Entry into the bursa is accomplished by use of the shaver/electrodiathermy.

Technical Tips

- Triangulation; practice with models and arthroscopic training courses.
- Excess bleeding or "red out."
    - Ensure irrigation fluid switched on and bag not empty or suction bottle full.
    - Ensure request for hypotensive anesthesia is enacted.
    - Stop/reduce fluid inflow to allow clotting or contracture of the vessel.
    - Increase fluid pressure/throughput. Perversely this may exacerbate the bleeding from the Bernoulli effect.
    - Diathermy to cauterize the vessel.
    - Ensure drainage through cannula or shaver not blocked.

Extra Portals

- The structures to avoid when adding working portals are the axillary nerve and the brachial plexus/neurovascular bundle. This allows a wide access for procedures such as stabilization by repair of the glenoid labrum and capsular placation.
- In effect, addition portals should NOT be inserted below the tendon of subscapularis anteriorly or infraspinatus posteriorly.
- Named portals include the Neviaser portal which passes medial to the acromion arch posterior to the clavicle. This portal passes through the rotator cuff, but allows direct access to the superior labrum.

Establishing Portals

- Portals can be established using an outside–in or inside–out technique.
- Accurate placement of a portal facilitates subsequent surgery.
- The author prefers to use a "switching stick" technique (Fig. 3.11a, b) where the arthroscope is

pushed against the capsule at the site of the desired position of the portal. The arthroscope is removed from the cannula, and a metal rod passed along the cannula and through the capsule to the skin. An incision is made over the tip of the rod, and a trocar with cannula passed over the rod into the joint. Care must be taken not to scrape the articular cartilage as some modern cannulae have very sharp edges.

Postoperative Treatment

- A collar cuff protection is often necessary for the first week.
- Physiotherapy, if necessary, is related with the pathology indentified.

Follow-up

- It is suggested that the patient to be followed for the next 2 and 4 weeks, and then, according to the pathology, indentified to be referred to a specialized clinic.

Further Reading

Bahu MJ, Trentacosta N, Vorys GC, et al. Multidirectional instability: evaluation and treatment options. Clin Sports Med. 2008;27(4):671–89.

Carter CW, Moros C, Ahmad CS, et al. Arthroscopic anterior shoulder instability repair: techniques, pearls, pitfalls, and complications. Instr Course Lect. 2008;57:125–32.

Dobson M, Cobiella C, Lee M. Traumatic anterior shoulder instability: current concepts in management. Br J Hosp Med (Lond). 2009;70(5):260–5.

Feeley BT, Gallo RA, Craig EV. Cuff tear arthropathy: current trends in diagnosis and surgical management. J Shoulder Elbow Surg. 2009;18(3):484–94.

Kropf EJ, Tjoumakaris FP, Sekiya JK. Arthroscopic shoulder stabilization: is there ever a need to open? Arthroscopy. 2007;23(7):779–84.

Acromioplasty

Roger Hackney

Indications

- Subacromial impingement which has failed to respond to conservative measures.
- Small degenerative rotator cuff tears up to 1 cm in diameter.

Pre-operative Planning

Clinical Assessment

- Restriction of overhead activity limited by pain rather than weakness.
- Night pain.
- Difficulty with activities of daily living such as dressing, caring for hair, and driving.
- Loss of last few degrees of forward flexion.
- Painful arc in abduction typically between 90 and 120°.
- Crescendo arc to 180° may indicate acromioclavicular joint involvement. Confirm by direct palpation of the AC joint and by reproducing pain by cross arm adduction.
- Positive impingement tests.
- Pain on stressing supraspinatus.
- Beware of young (under 30) or athletic individuals who may have a primary instability and secondary impingement. Assess for SLAP- and GH-joint instability.

Radiological Assessment

- Plain X-ray may show evidence of impingement changes of the greater tuberosity and undersurface of the acromion. Acromioclavicular joint osteoarthritis also shown (Fig. 4.1).
- Ultrasound scan in appropriate hands will show impingement dynamically with evidence of subacromial bursitis and bunching of the bursa on abduction. Also excludes rotator cuff tears.
- MRI scan is more expensive and not dynamic. It is unreliable in detecting rotator cuff tears without the

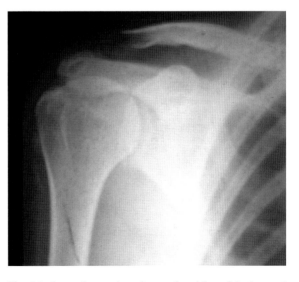

Fig. 4.1 Loss of space is a picture of upriding of the humeral head secondary to a massive cuff tear in a plain x-ray

R. Hackney
Department of Trauma and Orthopaedic Surgery,
Leeds Teaching Hospitals NHS Trust,
Leeds, UK
e-mail: roger.hackney@leedsth.nhs.uk

Fig. 4.2 (a) Typical bursal view findings of subacromial impingement. (b) The electrocautery device (*D*) clearing the subacromial bursa

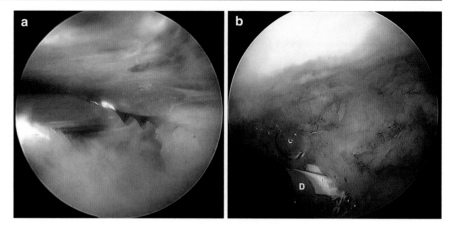

addition of an arthrogram. Arthrogram has been shown not to influence the procedure undertaken in the hands of an upper limb surgeon.

Operative Treatment

Anesthesia

- Regional (interscalene block) and/or general anesthesia.
- Hypotensive, systolic blood pressure below 100 mmHg.
- Antibiotic prophylaxis required if implants used

Table – Patient Positioning - Equipment

Beach chair, see (Fig. 3.2a):
- Use of Head ring or table support such as Schlein, see (Fig. 3.2b).
  Arthroscope with high flow cannula
- Camera stack system with light source, high definition television screen, photograph/video recording system for images (Fig. 3.4a).
- Arthroscopic pump and shaver, see (Fig. 3.4b).
- Electrocautery.
- Arthroscopic instruments, see (Fig. 3.5a–c).

Draping and Surgical Approach

- As per the diagnostic shoulder arthroscopy chapter, including a full inspection of the glenohumeral joint for comorbidities.

Acromioplasty

- The site of the lateral working portal for bursoscopy is 1 cm posterior to the anterolateral corner of the acromion. The sulcus between the acromion, and the humeral head is palpated and exaggerated by inferior traction on the arm. The scalpel blade is introduced parallel to the anterior edge of the acromion with a vertical incision.
- The trocar is introduced and triangulation skills used to position the tip of the trocar in front of the tip of the arthroscope. The surgical instrument is then positioned likewise.
- The relative position of the arthroscope is identified by observing the angle and position of the arthroscope. The position relative to the anterior and lateral acromion which lies outside the bursa is found by inserting a white gauge needle into the bursa space at the anterolateral corner of the acromion. A second white needle into the acromioclavicular joint marks the medial limit of the acromioplasty.
- Notice the typical bursal view findings of subacromial impingement (Fig. 4.2a).
- A soft-tissue shaver or electrocautery device with suction is introduced via the lateral portal. The author's preference is to use suction diathermy as this reduces the bleeding which can obscure the view (Fig. 4.2b).
- Wide sweeps of the operating arm are used to clear the subacromial bursa and demarcate the anterior and lateral edges of the acromion. The needles can be used as a guide to position within the bursa.
- The coracoacromial ligament is released from the acromion and divided.

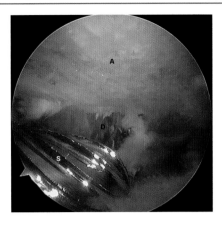

Fig. 4.3 The bony resection is performed with the deltoid attachment just visible (*A* acromion, *D* deltoid, *S* shaver)

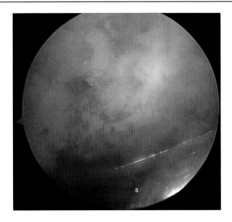

Fig. 4.4 Excision of lateral end of clavicle and full clearance observed (*S* shaver)

- A bone shaver is then used to smooth the acromion down to the level of origin of the deltoid muscle (Fig. 4.3).

Calcific Deposits

- Calcific tendinopathy is a common incidental finding on plain radiograph and other scanning modalities.
- Unless it is directly involved in the impingement process, then it is the author's practice to leave intratendinous deposits alone.
- If they are implicated by direct impingement and can be observed bulging through the tendon, then a needle can be used to make a fine incision in the tendon overlying the calcium.
- The deposit is commonly the consistency of cream cheese and can be removed by a soft-tissue shaver.

Excision Lateral End of Clavicle

- An additional anterior portal is introduced directly anterior and inferior to the acromioclavicular joint. The white needle can be used to locate the joint.
- A soft-tissue resector/diathermy is used to remove the AC joint capsule around the entire lateral end of the clavicle.
- The bone shaver is then used to remove the lateral 0.5 cm of the clavicle (Fig. 4.4).

- The entire rim of the bony cortex must be observed as a common technical error is to leave a superior overhang of bone, which will lead to persisting impingement and pain.

Postoperative Rehabilitation

- A polysling is worn for comfort until the interscalene block has worn off and for protection if out of the house for up to 2 weeks.
- Recovery and return to work is expected between 2 and 8 weeks depending upon occupation.
- Recent studies have shown that a home exercise program is as effective as attending formal physiotherapy sessions. The basic principles are that range of motion is restored passively using techniques, such as use of a pulley over a door or broom stick. Active range-of-motion work including climbing the hand up a wall. Strengthening work includes isometric training and use of theraband. Progression is tailored to the individual patient, it is important that the patient does not experience significant pain during the rehabilitation.

Follow-up

- The patient will be followed at the outpatient clinic for the following 2, 4, and 8 weeks.

Extra Tips

Open Versus Arthroscopic Acromioplasty

- Arthroscopic, able to inspect the shoulder joint for comorbidity, e.g., SLAP lesions, instability lesions, loose bodies, injury to articular cartilage, all of which may mimic subacromial impingement.
- The deltoid muscle is not damaged in the access to the subacromial space.
- The arthroscopic procedure is quicker, less painful, more easily undertaken as day case surgery, and the return to function in terms of work and sport is far more rapid.

Authors Comment

- In the opinion of the author, open arthroscopic decompression is a historical procedure which should not be undertaken by an upper limb surgeon.

Further Reading

Barfield LC, Kuhn JE. Arthroscopic versus open acromioplasty: a systematic review. Clin Orthop Relat Res. 2007;455:64–71.

Chin PY, Sperling JW, Cofield RH, et al. Anterior acromioplasty for the shoulder impingement syndrome: long-term outcome. J Shoulder Elbow Surg. 2007;16(6):697–700.

Neer CS2nd. Anterior acromioplasty for the chronic impingement in the shoulder. J Bone Joint Surg Am. 2005;87(6):1399.

Odenbring S, Wagner P, Atroshi I. Long-term outcomes of arthroscopic acromioplasty for chronic shoulder impingement syndrome: a prospective cohort study with a minimum of 12 years' follow-up. Arthroscopy. 2008;24(10):1092–8.

Rotator Cuff Repair (Open/Arthroscopic)

5

Roger Hackney

Introduction

- Open versus arthroscopic repair.
- Open repair involves disrupting the deltoid muscle. Repair is via per-osseous sutures to a bony trough.
- Arthroscopic repair of even large tears can be achieved with two portals, minimizing deltoid injury. Repair is via suture anchors. Double-row anchor techniques provide a footprint repair.
- Arthroscopic rotator cuff repair has results comparable to open repair, but has the advantages of less damage to deltoid, less pain, smaller scars, more rapid recovery with fewer adhesions, and in experienced hands the surgery is quicker. In addition, any other intra-articular pathology can be dealt with.

Preoperative Planning

Clinical Assessment

- Night pain.
- Weakness.
- Loss of overhead activity.
- Loss of function of activities of daily living.

R. Hackney
Department of Trauma and Orthopaedic Surgery,
Leeds Teaching Hospitals NHS Trust,
Leeds, UK
e-mail: roger.hackney@leedsth.nhs.uk

Examination

- Muscle wasting.
- Very variable from mild painful arc through to a flail shoulder.

Radiological Assessment

- Plain radiograph may show a number of changes (Fig. 5.1).
  - Up-riding of the humeral head measured against the glenoid.
  - The greater tuberosity and undersurface acromion may show:
    Mild subchondral sclerosis.
    Cyst formation.

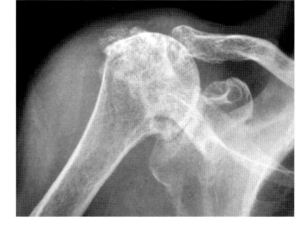

Fig. 5.1 X-ray of a patient with rotator cuff arthropathy

Acetabularization of the under-surface of the acromion.
- Rotator cuff arthropathy, "Milwaukee shoulder."
- Acromioclavicular joint osteoarthritis.
• Ultrasound scan (USS)
  - Size of tear, whether full or partial thickness.
  - Changes on articular or bursal side.
  - Impingement.
  - Bursitis.
  - Acromioclavicular joint changes.
• MRI arthrogram
  - Will show size of tear, but invasive and expensive compare with USS.
• CT/MRI scan may be very useful in the presence of significant muscle wasting to obtain the Goutallier score. This grades the degree of muscle atrophy by fatty infiltration. Greater than 50%, grades 3–4 give a much poorer result compared with grades 1–2.

Consideration for Surgery

• Discuss the options with the patient; conservative, simple sub-acromial decompression and rotator cuff repair.
• Take into account biological age and expectations of the patient, the size of the tear, the degree of muscle atrophy/fatty infiltration, social factors, and patient compliance.
• There is a risk of re-rupture greater with larger tears and older patients.
• There is no fixed age beyond which rotator cuff repair should not be undertaken as good results have been reported in 80-year olds.
• Small degenerative tears (>1 cm) can go into a watch and wait program if conservative treatment succeeds.

Open Rotator Cuff Repair

Anesthesia

• General anesthesia with interscalene block.
• Hypotensive anesthesia with systolic at or below 100 mmHg.

Table and Equipment

• Beach chair position with head secured in neutral position. Mayfield head ring or Schlein table attachment.
• Retractors for protecting deltoid.

Draping

• The arm is prepared with the forequarter.
• A U-drape placed around the upper chest/back, the hand is covered by a stockinet.

Incision

• The deltoid must be protected and preserved. Failure to adequately preserve deltoid causes considerable dysfunction of the shoulder.
• A lateral deltoid splitting approach is preferred. The incision is based 1–2 cm posterior to the anterior edge of the acromion and extends over the acromioclavicular joint. The distal extent is 4 cm from the lateral edge of the acromion approximately three patient fingers.
• Deltoid is split along the length of the incision with scissors.
• Care must be taken to avoid the axillary nerve which is usually at least 5 cm from the lateral acromion. The distal end of the deltoid split is protected from further extension by a Vicryl suture across deltoid.
• The anterolateral deltoid is then raised subperiosteally from the acromion.
• The subacromial bursa is exposed and removed, exposing the underlying rotator cuff.
• The undersurface of the anterolateral acromion is palpated and a subacromial decompression performed.
• A saw is used to remove about a third of the thickness of the undersurface of the acromion over the anterolateral 2 cm.
• The rotator cuff tear is identified (Fig. 5.2a) and the edges of the tear held with 2 ethibond stay sutures. The cuff is then released from any bursal adhesions using a finger or a pair of curved Mayo scissors (Fig. 5.2b). A release can extend as far as the spine of the scapula posteriorly and around the coracoid anteriorly. Release of the capsule from around the glenoid gives extra length when required. Gradual

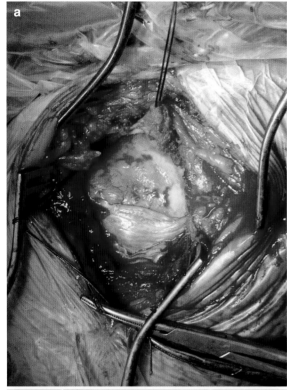

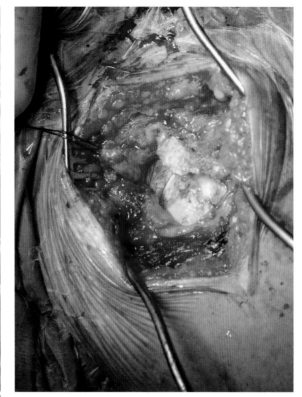

Fig. 5.3   The shape of the cuff tear is then assessed

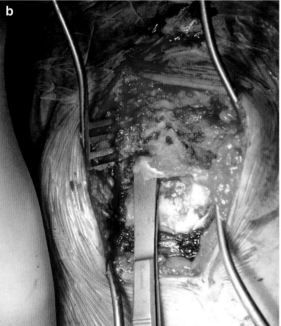

Fig. 5.2 (a) The rotator cuff tear is evident and the humeral head is exposed and often with cartilage defects. Suture placement at the rotator cuff. (b) Cuff is released from any bursal adhesions

release is achieved while applying traction through the stay sutures as the dissection progresses.

- The shape of the cuff tear is then assessed. A variety of shapes of tear are described (Fig. 5.3), but the key decision when repairing a tear is to pull the stay sutures together to determine how much of the repair should be from side to side sutures and how much from traction to re-attach to the tuberosities.
- Reattachment to the tuberosities is via per-osseous 5 ethibond sutures. A bone trough big enough to allow the edge of the cuff to be buried below the cortex is made just distal to the articular surface of the humeral head. The placement of these sutures distally should be below the tuberosity, roughly the length of arc of curvature of the needle. A bone awl may be required to penetrate the humeral shaft; the needle is then passed, and passed through the tendon. A Mason-Allen suture has the strongest hold on the tendon. The return suture should be per-osseous and pass out of the humeral shaft at least 1 cm from the first pass. Where more than

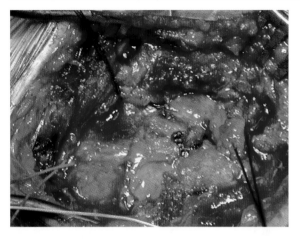

Fig. 5.4 Rotator cuff is repaired usually with ethibond N:5 sutures

one suture is used, the second hole from the first suture can be used for the first limb of the second.
- The rotator cuff is then repaired by sequentially tying the side to side sutures and then the perosseous sutures (Fig. 5.4). Additional sutures may be used passed through bone and tied over the top of the tendon to avoid any prominence from folds in the tendon.
- Deltoid is repaired fastidiously over the acromion. In older patients where the periosteal layer is thin, perosseous sutures through the acromion may be used.

Postoperative

- The arm is immobilized in a polysling in abduction for 6 weeks.
- Postoperative stiffness is reduced by gentle passive movements of the shoulder.
- Pendular exercises in and out of the sling plus passive movement below shoulder height are permitted.
- At 6 weeks, the patient is weaned from the shoulder and passive movements are replaced by passive-assisted motion prior to full active movement.

Follow-up

- It is related with the size of the rotator cuff tear and the operation performed.
- An appointment must be given in relation with sling removal (4–6 weeks).

- Physiotherapy is necessary afterward, and it is advisable to assess the patient regularly to evaluate effectiveness of physiotherapy.
- Time of recovery is dependent upon the size of tear, the age of the patient and the degree of muscle wasting, and ranges from 6 weeks to 6 months after removal of the sling.

Arthroscopic Rotator Cuff Repair

Anesthesia

- Hypotensive, systolic <100 mmHg.
- General anesthesia with interscalene block.

Table

- As per shoulder arthroscopy, Spider shoulder holder, e.g., TM Smith and Nephew.

Equipment

- Cannulae.
- Suction diathermy, rotator cuff repair instruments, e.g., express-sew TM Mitek, and elite instruments TM Smith and Nephew.
- Shaver, for subacromial decompression if required.
- Preferred suture anchors.

Technical Tips

- Arthroscopic rotator cuff repair requires advanced arthroscopic skills. Attendance at a course is a basic requirement, but ideally learning through a fellowship placement. Learn and practice the steps required. Practice basic techniques including knot tying on models.
- Make portals which fit the configuration of the tear.
- Use as many portals as necessary.
- Apply traction on the arm to achieve sufficient sub-acromial space. Sub-acromial decompression is occasionally required to obtain sufficient space (Fig. 5.5a, b).
- Fluid management, for control of bleeding, but avoid excess extravasation of fluid.

Fig. 5.5 (**a**) Sub-acromial decompression. (**b**) Synovitis associated with cuff tear (*A* acromion, *D* deltoid) (*S* synovitis, *LHB* long head of biceps, *H* humeral head)

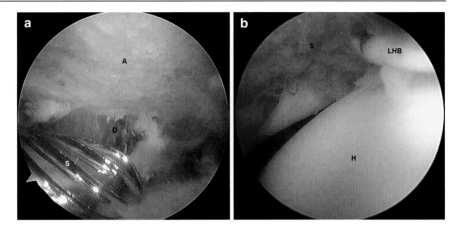

Fig. 5.6 (**a**) Debridement of bursa in a patient with rotator cuff tear (*D* diathermy, *B* bursa). (**b**) Bursal view of tear. Removing synovitis with diathermy (*D* diathermy, *s* synovitis)

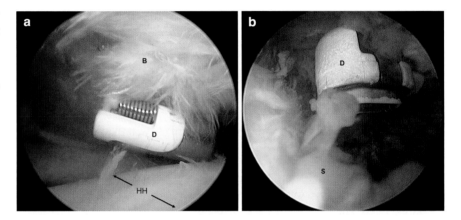

Fig. 5.7 (**a**) Suture placement (*RCT* rotator cuff tear, *S* suture). (**b**) Tighteninng suture in cuff tear (*RC* rotator cuff)

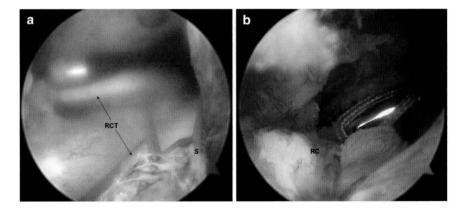

- It is possible to mobilize the tendon by removing bursal adhesions from around the coracoid process and spine of the scapula (Fig. 5.6a, b). The author prefers the use of suction diathermy to reduce bleeding.
- Traction sutures can be placed to determine the pattern of repair. Side-to-side sutures will close sizeable defects (Fig. 5.7a, b).

- Familiarize yourself with a small number of items of equipment from the vast number on the market, and practice techniques to mobilize and repair the tendon.
- Anchors are placed down the greater tuberosity, the area to which the tendon is repaired is debrided with a shaver.

- Simple sutures placed beyond the side to side sutures provide ample strength.
- Although confirmatory evidence is currently lacking it seems logical to obtain a footprint repair. There are a variety of techniques for this, but the simplest is to use the Quick T anchor TM Smith and Nephew, placed through the cuff once the lateral row of sutures has been placed.
- Check the repair from the articular side to ensure complete repair, and assess whether the repair is watertight.
- As part of the learning curve, the surgeon may wish to confirm the integrity of the repair with a mini-open incision. This also allows the surgeon to compare the arthroscopic and macroscopic appearances.
- Subscapularis repairs are the most difficult to accomplish, and the learning curve includes conversion to open repair.
- Subacromial decompression is not absolutely necessary, but usual.

Post Operative Rehabilitation

- Small tears require immobilization for 4 weeks in a polysling, larger tears 6 weeks.
- During this period, the shoulder is kept mobile with passive exercises at home and with the physiotherapist.
- Range of motion and isometric work begins after removal of the sling.

Follow-up

- Depending from the size of the rotator cuff tear and the operation performed.

- An appointment must be given in relation with sling removal (4–6 weeks).
- Physiotherapy is necessary afterward and it is advisable to assess the patient regularly to evaluate physiotherapy effectiveness.
- Time of recovery is dependent upon the size of tear, the age of the patient and the degree of muscle wasting, and ranges from 6 weeks to 6 months after removal of the sling.

Further Reading

Favard L, Bacle G, Berhouet J. Rotator cuff repair. Joint Bone Spine. 2007;74(6):551–7.

Labbé MR. Arthroscopic technique for patch augmentation of rotator cuff repairs. Arthroscopy. 2006;22(10):1136.e1–6.

Marx RG, Koulouvaris P, Chu SK, et al. Indications for surgery in clinical outcome studies of rotator cuff repair. Clin Orthop Relat Res. 2009;467(2):450–6.

Oh LS, Wolf BR, Hall MP, et al. Indications for rotator cuff repair: a systematic review. Clin Orthop Relat Res. 2007; 455:52–63.

Wolf BR, Dunn WR, Wright RW. Indications for repair of full-thickness rotator cuff tears. Am J Sports Med. 2007; 35(6):1007–16.

Saridakis P, Jones G. Outcomes of single-row and double-row arthroscopic rotator cuff repair: a systematic review. J Bone Joint Surg Am. 2010;92(3):732–42.

MacDonald PB, Altamimi S. Principles of arthroscopic repair of large and massive rotator cuff tears. Instr Course Lect. 2010;59:269–80.

Adla DN, Rowsell M, Pandey R. Cost-effectiveness of open versus arthroscopic rotator cuff repair. J Shoulder Elbow Surg. 2010;19(2):258–61.

Open Anterior Shoulder Stabilization

David Limb

Indications

- Recurrent dislocation or symptoms of instability after dislocation.
- In young people, the risk of recurrent dislocation after an index dislocation is very high, and some would consider stabilization after a single dislocation, particularly in those younger than 20 years of age.
- However, there is some evidence that there may be an increased risk of degenerative change on long-term review if this protocol is followed, and this cannot be considered to be an absolute indication.
- It should go without saying that anterior stabilization is for anterior instability, so care has to be taken to ensure that there is not a major posterior or inferior element to the instability pattern.

Preoperative Planning

Clinical Assessment

- There is a history of anterior dislocation with further episodes of dislocation, or a recurring sense of insecurity when the arm is used in abduction and external rotation.

D. Limb
Leeds General Infirmary,
Leeds, UK
e-mail d.limb@leeds.ac.uk

- It is unusual for there to be any wasting or limitation of movement. Deltoid wasting should alert to the possibility of axillary nerve injury.
- Apprehension tests are positive in most cases. A combination of apprehension in abduction and external rotation that is eased by posteriorly directed pressure over the humeral head is good evidence for anterior instability.
- Tests for multidirectional laxity (e.g., the presence of a sulcus sign when downward traction is exerted on the arm when it is on the side) should be negative – if not then the case is more complex and anterior stabilization should not be carried out without further investigation and assessment.

Radiological Assessment

- AP and axial views of the shoulder may be normal. However, there is commonly evidence of a Hill Sachs lesion – an impaction fracture of the posterior aspect of the humeral head created by pressure from the anterior glenoid rim when the shoulder is dislocated forward.
- A very large Hill Sachs lesion should alert to the possibility of the edge of the lesion engaging on the anterior glenoid rim in abduction and external rotation. This can produce dislocation in itself and can disrupt repairs, so should cause one to consider non-anatomic anterior stabilization, for example, using a Latarjet procedure (transfer of the coracoid process and its attached conjoint tendon to the anterior glenoid rim).

- CT or MR arthrography can give useful information on the anatomy of the lesion causing instability. This is important as repairs should aim to restore normal anatomy. They can also identify any deficiency of the glenoid that may need grafting, CT being easier to reconstruct in 3D.
- Many surgeons would not use investigations of this sort for straightforward cases of recurrent anterior dislocation, but instead proceed to arthroscopy, which allows examination under anesthesia and visualization of the ligament and capsule lesions and inspection of any bony lesions. It also allows the surgeon to proceed directly to repair either through the arthroscope or as an open procedure. Arthroscopy is not as good as CT, however, for accurate study of bone lesions.

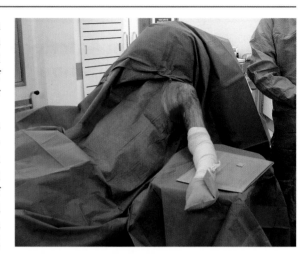

Fig. 6.1 The beach chair position

Operative Technique

Anesthesia

- Regional anesthesia, using an interscalene block, enables shoulder arthroscopy and either open or arthroscopic stabilization to be carried out with the patient awake. It relies on the necessary skills being available but, nowadays, particularly with ultrasound to aid placement of the needle tip, is increasingly reliable.
- General anesthesia is an alternative, while many prefer to use an interscalene block for analgesia while taking advantage of a light general anesthetic to avoid problems with positioning, draping, and patient movement.
- With the prolonged effect of regional blocks, it is usually possible to carry out open shoulder stabilization as a day-case procedure in much the same way that arthroscopic procedures are.

Positioning and Equipment

- The beach chair position is ideal for open shoulder stabilization (Fig. 6.1).
- If arthroscopy is carried out beforehand, then it is preferred that the arthroscopy is also carried out in the beach chair position to avoid the need to reposition the patient between procedures.
- Basic surgical instruments are required for the approach and closure, including self-retaining retractors.

- Specialized shoulder retractors greatly facilitate exposure of the glenoid and allow access using a small incision. Self-retaining retractors with interchangeable blades allow a deep blade to be placed medially under the conjoint tendon, while a shallower blade holds the deltoid away from the field.
- Inside the shoulder joint, a Fukuda, or similar ring retractor, holds the humeral head laterally and backward exposing the glenoid rim and labrum anteriorly.
- Spiked retractors can be placed beneath subscapularis onto the anterior surface of the glenoid neck, further facilitating the view of the anterior glenoid rim and labrum.
- A means of reconstructing the anterior labral attachment to the glenoid, or rebuilding a bone deficiency of the glenoid itself, is needed. Tissue anchors are usually used for soft-tissue repairs, while a small fragment set allows attachment of bone grafts or the transposed coracoid process to the anterior glenoid. If the labral attachment is not pathological, then sutures alone may be used for capsular shift or capsulolabral reconstruction.

Surgical Approach

- A standard deltopectoral approach can be used; it gives good access to the shoulder joint, and may be needed if a Latarjet procedure is to be carried out or if an iliac crest bone graft is used to reconstruct an anterior glenoid bone deficiency.

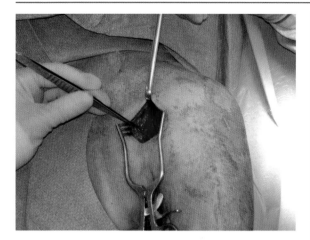

Fig. 6.2 The cephalic vein is identified to locate the deltopectoral groove

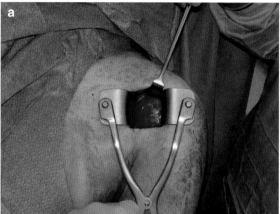

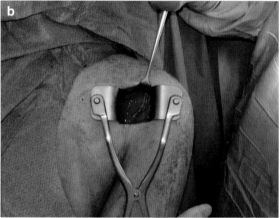

Fig. 6.3 (**a**) The self retaining retractor is placed beneath deltoid and the conjoint tendon to expose subscapularis. (**b**) Subscapularis is divided leaving the capsule beneath intact and a cuff of tendon laterally for reattachment. The inferior third of the tendon can be left completely intact

- For an open Bankart procedure, inferior capsular, capsulolabral reconstruction or similar soft-tissue reconstruction, a much smaller incision can be used, still taking advantage of the deltopectoral interval.
- With the arm by the side, the anterior axillary crease is noted. The arm is then abducted slightly and a 4–5-cm incision is made along the line of the anterior axillary fold. This gives excellent cosmesis afterward.
- The cephalic vein is identified and retracted laterally with the deltoid as the deltopectoral interval is opened (Fig. 6.2). There is often a small arterial branch crossing the surgical field from the region of the coracoid to the deltoid, which can be divided after controlling for bleeding.
- The thoracobrachial fascia is thus exposed and is opened along the lateral margin of the conjoint tendon. A deep retractor blade is placed beneath the tendon, while a shallower blade is placed under deltoid – these are attached to a self-retaining retractor which is then used to open the surgical field to expose the subscapularis tendon (Fig. 6.3a).

The Surgical Procedure

- This description will now focus on the open Bankart repair, as at this point the various methods of stabilization deviate, and the way that the subscapularis tendon is breached differs between procedures.
- The subscapularis tendon is divided, leaving the underlying capsule intact. This is facilitated by

holding the arm in external rotation, but can still be very difficult! (Fig. 6.3b).
- The subscapularis tendon and capsule are intimately fused laterally, while the subscapularis muscle is easily dissected away from the underlying capsule medially. However, if the subscapularis is divided at its myotendinous junction, a secure repair cannot be effected at the end. Furthermore, a capsular shift is much more limited if only the medial extent of the capsule is exposed.
- The author prefers to leave approximately 1 cm of subscapularis attached to the lesser tuberosity. By dividing carefully through this the transition between silvery, horizontally oriented collagen fibers of tendon and the more amorphous yellowish

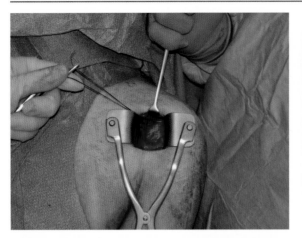

Fig. 6.4 The capsule is exposed after carefully dissecting off the subscapularis tendon

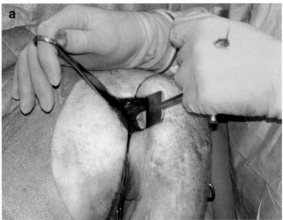

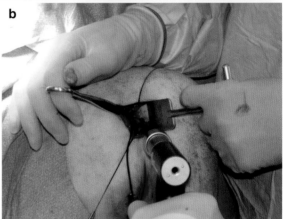

Fig. 6.5 (**a**) The Fukuda retractor is placed to retract the humeral head and exposed the anterior glenoid rim from which the labrum has been avulsed. (**b**) Drilling for anchor placement

capsule can be identified and the dissection turned medially in this plane.

- Furthermore approximately one third of the subscapularis tendon can be left intact inferiorly – this allows a secure repair and is excellent for gauging the anatomical site of repair at the end (Fig. 6.3b). Since the muscle fibers of subscapularis extend closer to the humeral attachment inferiorly, the correct interval is more quickly reached at the bottom of the surgical transgression through subscapularis and can be used to guide tendon and capsule separation upward until the rotator interval is reached.
- The upper two thirds of subscapularis can then be retracted medially with stay sutures, exposing the capsule.
- The capsule is opened in a way that facilitates closure incorporating a capsular shift – a traumatic avulsion of the labrum often stretches or tears capsule, and this redundancy needs to be dealt with (Fig. 6.4).
- A sideway's "T" capsulotomy gives excellent access to the joint. The vertical limb can be medial or lateral, the author preferring the latter, as described in Neer's paper on the inferior capsular shift. Stay sutures are placed in the apices of the two medial capsular flaps that are thus created. The inferior flap is gently lifted upward, and the vertical limb extended down to the axillary recess, taking up any capsular redundancy.
- A Fukuda retractor is placed in the glenohumeral joint and used to retract the humeral head and expose the labrum (Fig. 6.5a). A spiked retractor

medially onto the glenoid neck completes exposure of the labrum.

- The separated labrum is identified, and the glenoid prepared for reattachment using a rasp to scarify the bone surface. If the labrum has reattached onto the scapular neck, it has to be mobilized to enable reattachment to create an anterior buffer on the glenoid rim.
- Anchors are placed in the glenoid rim (Fig. 6.5b) – the number used will depend on the extent of reattachment required. Anchors 5 mm or closer together are probably too close while anything over 1 cm is probably too far apart.
- The lower anchor is usually at the level of attachment of the anterior band of the inferior glenohumeral ligament. After placing the anchor, the labrum and ligaments are lifted up to guage where they should sit on the glenoid. The sutures attached

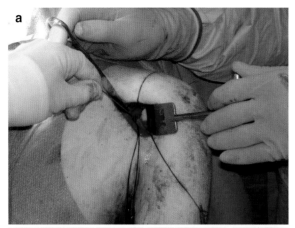

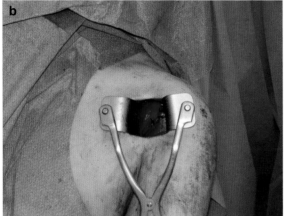

Fig. 6.6 (**a**) The sutures are tied to repair the labrum and capsule to the glenoid rim. (**b**) The subscapularis is repaired with no. 2 sutures to its anatomical position

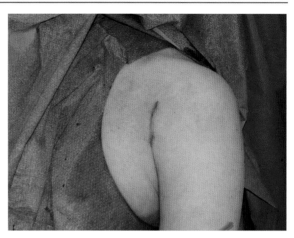

Fig. 6.7 The skin wound is closed with an absorbable suture and the scar is in line with the anterior axillary fold for improved cosmesis

- With the arm in external rotation the capsular flaps are overlapped to take up any slack, resulting in a double-breasting effect of the anterior capsule in most cases. However, the capsule is not put under tension during repair and sometimes simple anatomical closure is all that is required to take up any slack.
- On removal of the retractors, the deltopectoral interval falls back together. Absorbable fat sutures are placed before subcuticular skin closure (Fig. 6.7).
- A polysling or similar shoulder immobilizer is applied.

to the anchor are passed through the labrum and capsule at the relevant point, and retrieved from beneath the subscapularis.

- Once tied, the space for suture placement and needle handling in the joint quickly becomes restricted, so it is usual to place all the anchors and pass the sutures out through the labrum and capsule before tying the sutures, starting at the important inferior anchor and working up (Fig. 6.6a).
- After repair of the anterior labrum, recreating a buffer on the anterior glenoid, the capsule can be closed. The arm is placed in 30° of external rotation before capsular closure to ensure there is no restriction of rotation after surgery.
- Closure of the rotator interval is also carried out before suturing the capsule, as the interval can be pulled open by excessive overlap of the capsule (Fig. 6.6b).

Postoperative Care and Rehabilitation

- There are many and varied protocols for rehabilitation after arthroscopic and open-shoulder stabilization. They have not been rigorously compared in any scientific way, so use a method that is agreed among surgeon, patient, and therapists to avoid confusion.
- The author prefers that the operated arm is rested in the polysling for 1 week. The sling can then be discarded, and use of the arm for simple activities of daily living is allowed.
- Rehabilitation also begins at this point, though stretching or tensing the capsule and subscapularis repairs should be avoided initially.
- This can be achieved by avoiding external rotation of the arm past the neutral position or elevation of the humerus above horizontal for 3 months.

- This does not mean that the hand cannot be used overhead – with the humerus horizontal and the arm far short of the neutral position, the top of the head is easily reached.
- Full range of movement is allowed at 3 months and subscapularis strengthening begins. Of perhaps more importance, however, is restoration of the proprioceptive functions of the capsule.
- Contact sports and occupations that carry a high risk of the arm being wrenched into external rotation are commenced at 6 months.

Complications

- Theoretically, infection is a risk, but with a minimal approach and the inherently good blood supply of the shoulder, this is a rarity, but a disaster if it occurs.
- Enthusiastic retraction can risk damage to the musculocutaneous nerve, while dividing the inferior part of the subscapularis and inferior capsule risks injury to the axillary nerve.
- Stiffness is a risk after open repairs, though is not the inevitability that it was when the Putti Platt repair was standard. With modern anatomic repairs, the loss of movement should be a few degrees of external rotation only.
- Capsulitis can complicate any shoulder surgery; however, even if there have been no errors in judgment in closing the capsule. Fortunately, the full-blown syndrome of global stiffness seen in a frozen shoulder is rare, and is not specific to open stabilization.

Results

- Open stabilization using a Bankart repair for a Bankart lesion is the gold standard for shoulder stabilization, yet the precise figures for comparison are clouded.
- Historically, the procedure is reported to be successful in preventing redislocation in around 95% of patients.
- Recent comparisons with arthroscopic repair suggest that there is little difference in outcome between the procedures. However, open procedures tend to be selected for more difficult cases, many surgeons are no longer as familiar with open reconstruction, and most studies are underpowered with insufficient follow-up. It seems to be the norm to report results of stabilization 2 years after surgery, the assumption being that if further episodes of dislocation have not occurred by then, then they are unlikely to happen. However, the recurrences after open surgery that are reported often occur 5 years or more after the index procedure.
- Suffice it to say that the best operation is the one that the surgeon does best, and if there is still genuinely a choice to be made, then the patient should perhaps be involved in making that choice.

Follow-up

- The patient is regularly inspected at 2 weeks and the following 1, 3, and 6 months. Some surgeons prefer additional longer follow up at one and/or two years, particularly if they are involved in research or audit of their results.

Further Reading

Hobby J, Griffin D, Dunbar M, et al. Is arthroscopic surgery for stabilisation of chronic shoulder instability as effective as open surgery? A systematic review and meta-analysis of 62 studies including 3044 arthroscopic operations. J Bone Joint Surg Br. 2007;89(9):1188–96.

Khazzam M, Kane SM, Smith MJ. Open shoulder stabilization procedure using bone block technique for treatment of chronic glenohumeral instability associated with bony glenoid deficiency. Am J Orthop. 2009;38(7):329–35.

Langford J, Bishop J, Lee E, et al. Outcomes following open repair of Bankart lesions for recurrent, traumatic anterior glenohumeral dislocations. Orthopedics. 2006;29(11):1008–13.

Wolf BR, Strickland S, Williams RJ, et al. Open posterior stabilization for recurrent posterior glenohumeral instability. J Shoulder Elbow Surg. 2005;14(2):157–64.

Arthroscopic Shoulder Stabilization

7

Roger Hackney

Indications

- History of frank dislocation, recurrent dislocation, or subluxation with or without radiological support.
- Painful shoulder in overhead or contact athlete.
- First time dislocation under 23 years of age in a contact sport.

Preoperative Assessment

Clinical Assessment

- Positive apprehension and/or SLAP tests.
- Presence of hypermobility/excessive joint laxity.
- Examine the contralateral shoulder for external rotation with the elbow by the side and with the shoulder at 90° of abduction.
- Sulcus sign.
- Measure Beighton score.
- Scapular pseudowinging.
- Habitual or voluntary dislocators are treated with specialized rehabilitation.

Radiological Assessment

- Plain radiographs.
- Trauma views to confirm direction of instability.

7

R. Hackney
Department of Trauma and Orthopaedic Surgery,
Leeds Teaching Hospitals NHS Trust, Leeds, UK
e-mail roger.hackney@leedsth.nhs.uk

- Obtain views to exclude Hill–Sachs lesion, bony Bankart (Fig. 7.1a, b).
- CT scan is necessary to confirm size of bony lesions. If the bony lesion is large, the patients may be excluded from arthroscopic repair (Fig. 7.2).
- MRI arthrogram is expensive and unnecessary, as it is not sufficiently sensitive or specific to provide information which is not obtained by examination and arthroscopy.

Operative Treatment

- Open versus arthroscopic stabilization. Arthroscopic stabilization produces results comparable with the best open repairs. If anything the criteria for arthroscopic success are more stringent, as historically, the end point for success in open stabilization was recurrent dislocation. Arthroscopic stabilization is regarded as unsuccessful if instability symptoms persist even without frank dislocation.
- Arthroscopic stabilization is less painful, recovery is quicker, scars are smaller, but perhaps, more importantly, all aspects of instability can be addressed, and the experienced surgeon possesses a variety of techniques to cope with the many variants of glenohumeral joint instability. It can be used to dramatically reduce the risk of recurrence in young first-time dislocators in contact sports.
- Arthroscopic surgery is not suitable for those with significant bony injury, and some argue that high-energy contact-sport players are better served by a Latarjet procedure.

P.V. Giannoudis (ed.), *Practical Procedures in Elective Orthopaedic Surgery*,
DOI 10.1007/978-0-85729-820-1_7, © Springer-Verlag London Limited 2012

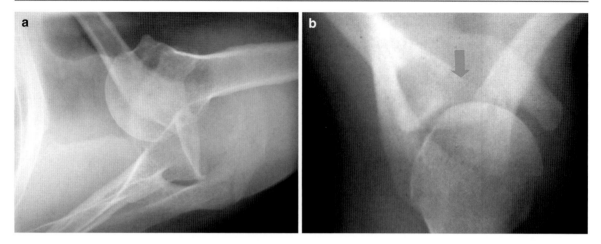

Fig. 7.1 (**a**) Anterior dislocation (*axillary view*). (**b**) X-ray of a bony bankart lesion (*arrow*)

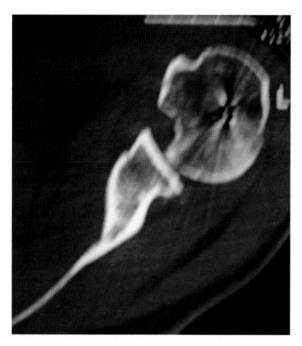

Fig. 7.2 Hill–Sachs lesion on CT

- There is a long learning curve and techniques should be learned on models and developed in specialist placements/fellowships. Knot tying requires constant practice.

Anesthesia

- General anesthesia with interscalene block.
- Hypotensive anesthesia.

Table Setup

- Instruments the same side as the surgeon within the clean air environment.

Patient Positioning

- Beach chair; use of head ring or table support, such as Schlein.
- Lateral position; lateral supports, traction equipment fixed to table.

Equipment

- All as per shoulder arthroscopy, with additional instruments for stabilization. This includes a means of releasing the capsule from the glenoid, a method of passing sutures through the capsule and suture anchors (Fig. 7.3).

Draping and Approach

- A careful examination of the shoulder under anesthetic is undertaken of BOTH shoulders. Range of motion and laxity are compared, and the degree of laxity/instability recorded in several variations of abduction and external rotation of the shoulder.

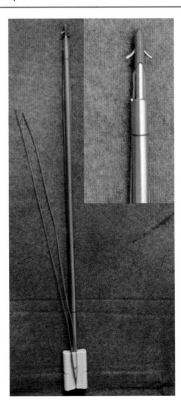

Fig. 7.3 Suture anchor

- A standard arthroscopic examination of the glenohumeral joint is undertaken (Fig. 7.4a). Care must be taken to assess the rotator cuff, the glenoid labrum and the inferior capsular attachment of the humeral head to exclude the HAGL lesion (Humeral Avulsion of Glenohumeral Ligament).
- The superior labrum is probed to assess stability (Fig. 7.4b).
- The presence of variants of anatomy, such as the sub-labral hole or Buford complex, is checked.
- The distance between the bare area in the middle of the glenoid articular surface and the glenoid edge at 5 and 7 o'clock is compared. If the anterior distance is less than 50% of the posterior measurement, then the patient is not suitable for an arthroscopic repair.
- If a Hill–Sachs lesion and/or bony Bankart lesion are found, the shoulder is placed in abduction and internal rotation to try to place the Hill–Sachs lesion against the edge of the glenoid. If this occurs, then the patient is not suitable for an arthroscopic repair, and an open procedure, such as a Latarjet, is recommended.

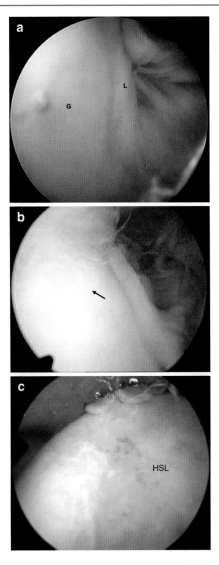

Fig. 7.4 (**a**) Normal glenoid (*G*) and labrum (*L*). (**b**) A type I SLAP lesion (*arrow*), (**c**) A Hill–Sachs lesion (*HSL*), indentified arthroscopicaly

Technique

- The usual finding is of a Bankart lesion in the lower half of the anterior glenoid. Also, the Hill–Sachs lesion could be detected (Fig. 7.4c). The labrum is detached from the edge of the glenoid and sags inferiorly.
- A second portal is established depending upon the position of the lesion. The portal must be sufficiently lateral to allow access for a drill onto the

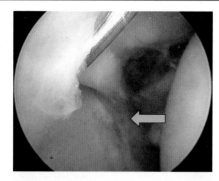

Fig. 7.5 A SLAP injury (*arrow*)

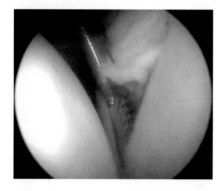

Fig. 7.6 A knife rasp is used to elevate the capsule from where it has healed to the glenoid

glenoid. A SLAP (Fig. 7.5) lesion will require a further working portal either through the rotator cuff tendon or the Neviaser portal. The site for the portal is gauged by use of a white needle.

- A knife rasp is used to elevate the capsule from where it has healed to the glenoid. (Fig. 7.6).
- The release is sufficient when the capsule sits back in an anatomical position.
- A grasper is used to elevate the capsule into the required position on the glenoid. The arm is then externally rotated to ensure that excess capsule has not been held by the grasper, if so, then the capsule will pull away from the glenoid. This technique is especially important when assessing Bankart lesions which extend to the upper half of the glenoid, thus avoiding "repairing" a sublabral hole.
- The neck of the glenoid is freshened using a knife rasp or arthroscopic shaver. The older the injury the more aggressive I am.

- There are a variety of techniques described to place an anchor in the glenoid and place sutures from the anchor through the required capsule. The surgeon should be practiced and familiarized with at least one of these methods.
- One such technique is described.
  - The position of the glenoid where the capsule reaches is noted, and the anchor position marked with a rongeur onto the anterior surface of the edge of the glenoid. The bone is exposed and freshened further, and a drill used to prepare the hole for the anchor. At least two anchors should be used, depending upon the size of the tear. The repair is undertaken from inferior to superior, except in the presence of a SLAP lesion which is repaired first.
  - A spectrum suture passer can be used to pass a "1" PDS thread through the required piece of capsule pushing an excess of thread into the joint. The spectrum instrument is removed leaving the suture through the capsule.
  - The intra-articular piece of suture is grabbed with a suture grasper, and pulled out through the same portal.
  - A Mitek G2 anchor is then threaded down the suture limb which has just been pulled out of the joint into the pre-drilled hole. The anchor delivery system is removed, leaving the orthocord (or orthocord replacement) on the anchor. A sliding knot is tied externally and the capsule tied down onto the glenoid. Three half-hitches are added for security. Care must be taken to ensure that each knot is snugged down onto the capsule. An instrument such an arthropierce is then passed though the capsule to grasp the ethibond thread and pull this back through the portal. A second sliding knot is tied secured by further half-hitches.
  - This is repeated as many times as indicated (Fig. 7.7). The capsule can be reefed medially and superiorly according to the findings on EUA and the arthroscopic assessment. The rotator interval may be broadened; it can be closed by a two portal technique using the spectrum system or with non-absorbable sutures using suture shuttle techniques and two working portals.

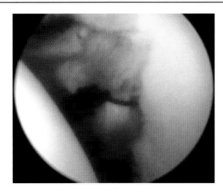

Fig. 7.7   The labral tear is repaired

– The shoulder is then carefully examined for external rotation and stability.

Postoperative Rehabilitation

• A polysling is worn for 3 weeks with passive movements of the shoulder permitted plus elbow range of motion exercises.

• Range of motion work is followed by strengthening exercises and progression to sports specific training.
• Most surgeons recommend at least 6 months avoidance of contact sports or exercise in an abducted and externally rotated position.

Follow-up

• Physiotherapy continuse for a 16 week programme. Out-patient follow is a 6-8 weeks and subsequent review if any clinical problems arise.

Further Reading

Bottoni CR, Smith EL, Berkowitz MJ, et al. Arthroscopic versus open shoulder stabilization for recurrent anterior instability: a prospective randomized clinical trial. Am J Sports Med. 2006;34(11):1730–7.

Hiemstra LA, Sasyniuk TM, Mohtadi NG, et al. Shoulder strength after open versus arthroscopic stabilization. Am J Sports Med. 2008;36(5):861–7.

Ogilvie-Harris DJ, D'Angelo G. Arthroscopic surgery of the shoulder. Sports Med. 1990;9(2):120–8.

Arthroscopic Capsular Release for Shoulder Stiffness

8

Arup K. Bhadra, Craig S. Roberts, and Frank O. Bonnarens

Introduction

- Shoulder stiffness can result due to primary idiopathic adhesive capsulitis or secondary to known intrinsic, extrinsic, or systemic conditions (including posttraumatic stiffness and postoperative stiffness).
- Primary idiopathic adhesive capsulitis
  - Considered a painful self-limiting disease that resolves after 1–3 years.
  - Incidence is estimated to be around 2–5% in the general population.
  - Women comprise approximately 70%.
  - Contralateral shoulder is likely to be involved in 20–30% of patients.
  - Pathology results from intraarticular inflammation and fibrosis which causes contracture of the capsule and a reduced intraarticular volume.
  - It is believed to result from a systemic disorder (inflammatory, endocrine, immunologic, biochemical), although a definite etiology is not known.
  - Hannafin and Chiaia described four stages of adhesive capsulitis:
    Stage 1: "Initial painful phase" (0–3 months) – pain with active and passive ROM, some limitation of movements

Stage 2: "Freezing stage" (3–9 months) – chronic pain with active and passive ROM, significant limitation of movements
Stage 3: "Frozen stage" (9–15 months) – minimal pain except at end ROM, significant limitation of ROM with rigid "end feel"
Stage 4: "Thawing stage" (15–36 months) – minimal pain, progressive improvement in ROM

- Secondary adhesive capsulitis can result in global loss of active and passive ROM or reduced ROM in specific plane depending on the etiology.
  - Asymmetric loss of motion results from scarring in the area affected
  - Contracture may be intraarticular or extraarticular.
  - Particular pattern of limitation in ROM can assist with planning rehabilitation protocol or particular operative management
  - Reduced external rotation in adduction suggests contractures of the anterosuperior capsule and the rotator interval
  - Loss of external rotation in abduction is associated with contractures of the anteroinferior capsule
  - Decreased internal rotation in abduction or adduction and reduced cross-chest adduction is indicative of posterior capsular contractures

A.K. Bhadra (✉) • C.S. Roberts • F.O. Bonnarens
Academic Department of Trauma and Orthopaedics,
School of Medicine,University of Louisville,
Louisville, KY, USA
e-mail: arupbhadra@yahoo.com

Clinical Presentation

- All type of adhesive capsulitis present with painful limited shoulder motion.
- Pain at rest and at night that is aggravated with extreme ROM is a common symptom.

- Routine activities of daily living that require reaching overhead or behind the back are painful and difficult.
- Patients demonstrate global restriction (less than 50% of that of contralateral side) of active and passive movements.

Evaluation and Diagnosis

- Numerous other shoulder conditions may present with painful and stiff shoulder.
- Detailed history, physical examination, and radiographic evaluation are important.
- Associated rotator cuff disease present with passive motion greater than active motion, weakness of involved muscles, and abnormal MRI scans or arthrograms.
- Detailed history of prior trauma or shoulder difficulties is important.
- Evaluation of cervical spine and endocrine system, e.g., diabetes, thyroid, etc. should be included in the examination.
- Both active and passive ROM should be documented. It is critical that compensatory mechanism such as shoulder shrugging, trunk lean, or scapulothoracic movements be corrected for. Passive ROM should be performed with the patient supine or by stabilizing the scapula with one hand.
- Standard AP, scapular lateral, and axillary radiographs may be normal in idiopathic adhesive capsulitis but can help reveal glenohumeral arthritis, fractures or malunions, loose bodies, calcific tendinitis, dislocations, hardware, and disuse osteopenia.
- MRI arthrogram is excellent for evaluating associated pathology, such as a rotator cuff tear. MRI is also helpful to delineate acromioclavicular joint arthropathy.

Arthroscopic Capsular Release

Indications

- Persistent shoulder pain and stiffness after 6 months of failed conservative care.
- If the shoulder pain is severe enough to awaken the patient every night or many times at night.

Table 8.1 Treatment options for adhesive capsulitis

• Benign neglect • Home exercise • Supervised physical therapy • NSAIDs • Intraarticular steriod injections • Distension arthrography-"Brisement procedure" • Closed manipulation under anesthetics • Arthroscopic capsular release • Open capsular release • Combination of above	Achieves remission 60–80% of cases

- Severe stiffness – 0° external rotation, 30° abduction, moderate stiffness – a decrease of 30° in either plane when compared with the contralateral side.
- If manipulation under anesthesia does not restore 80% of the ROM of the normal side.
- If at 6 months stiffness persists, but pain has diminished, it may be into the "thaw" phase and it is advisable to continue 2 more months with nonoperative care. Surgery should be considered if there is no improvement even after that.
- External rotation is the most important predictor of success or failure of conservative management. Persistent loss of external rotation at 4–6 months after the start of conservative care indicates a stiff shoulder less likely to respond to nonoperatve care, hence earlier operative intervention is indicated.
- Treatment options for adhesive capsulitis are presented at Table 8.1.

Contraindications

- Patients with extraarticular contracture, especially subscapularis shortening or contracture between subscapularis and conjoined tendon.
- Patients with previous internal fixation or severly malunited fractures which may need open surgery to remove the hardware or corrective osteotomy, respectively.
- Patients in the inflammatory or contracting phase of idiopathic adhesive capsulitis.

Anesthesia

- General anesthesia through an endotracheal tube with the tube oriented away from the affected shoulder.
- Interscalene block with or without an indwelling catheter using 0.5% bupivacaine with epinephrine (1: 200000).
- Perioperative prophylactic antibiotics.

Manipulation Under Anesthesia

- After induction of anesthesia, both shoulders are examined for ROM in supine position.
- Gentle manipulation of arm is performed in forward flexion to the maximum possible extent, after stabilizing the scapula with one hand.
- Next, passive external rotation is performed in 0° of abduction followed by 90° of abduction.
- Lastly, internal rotation is performed in 90° of abduction and cross-body adduction.
- If expected (80%) improvement in ROM is not achieved, arthroscopic surgery is performed.

Table and Equipment

- Routine shoulder arthroscopy instruments set with 30° 4.5-mm arthroscope, 3.5-mm motorized shavers, electrocautery device, 7-mm cannula.
- The instruments used more commonly are placed on a Mayo stand on the side of surgery (Fig. 8.1).

Patient Positioning

- Lateral decubitus or beach chair position as per surgeon's choice
  - Lateral decubitus:
    Patient is assisted on the table and centered on the beanbag
    Patient is turned over on the unaffected side
    Beanbag is gathered up around the patient and deflated until it is firm
    The operating table is tilted 20–30° posterior so that the glenoid is parallel to the floor
    Adequate padding around the pressure points is done to protect soft tissue and neurovascular structures

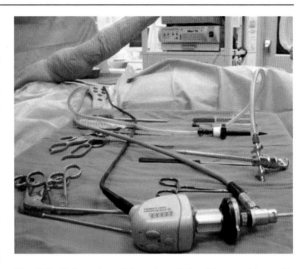

Fig. 8.1 Patient draped in a lateral decubitus position with routine shoulder arthroscopy instruments on a Mayo table on the surgeon's side

A rolled sheet is placed under upper thorax "axillary roll" to minimize pressure on neurovascular structure within the axilla
A suspension device is stabilized at the foot end of the table, the patient's shoulder is placed in 60° abduction and 10° flexion, and traction and stabilization of arm is done with 10–15 lbs of weight
  - Beach Chair position:
    Patient's thorax must be placed 70–80° upright to the floor
    Small amount of Trendelenburg positioning is applied; legs are lowered until the patient's acromion is almost parallel to the floor
    Pillows are placed under the knees and pressure points are protected

Draping

- Aseptic skin preparation of the shoulder and arm from the neck and lower border of mandible, mid-chest, axilla, and distally up to the wrist is performed.
- Two U-drapes are placed around the neck and axilla to create water-sealed operative field.
- Stockinette is secured around the hand and forearm and attached with the traction device, in case of lateral decubitus.
- A fluid collection pouch is applied around the axilla and at the back of the shoulder.

Surgical Technique

- Preoperative ROM is assessed by the surgeon once the patient is asleep and the muscle relaxation is achieved. Although formal manipulation is no longer performed, examinations of all arcs of motion starting with anterior flexion are performed. Once a soft endpoint is reached, gentle overpressure is used until there is a firm endpoint at which the ROM of that arc is stopped.
- An 18-gauge spinal needle is carefully introduced posteriorly over the humeral head into the joint and 10–20-mL sterile saline solution is injected to increase the glenohumeral space for safer introduction of the arthroscope (Fig. 8.2a).
- The arthroscope is introduced through the posterior portal through the conventional soft spot. The correct intraarticular placement is confirmed by backflow of fluid out of the arthroscope sheath.
- The arthroscope is directed towards the rotator interval. A spinal needle is inserted percutaneously lateral to the coracoid process and guided to enter the joint just underneath the biceps tendon (Fig. 8.2b).
- The spinal needle is replaced with a 7-mm cannula.
- Two types of release have been described: 180° release and 360° release. The latter involves releasing the entire capsule including the infraglenoid segment (5 o' clock to 7 o' clock position) which is intimately adjacent to the axillary nerve.

Anterior Capsular Release

- The first step is to release the rotator interval.
- A 3.5-mm motorized shaver is used to debride the inflamed synovium and scar tissue from an area bounded by the biceps tendon medially, by the superior border of subscapularis inferiorly, and by the humeral head laterally.
- The middle glenohumeral ligament is identified and separated from the superior border of subscapularis and released with an electrocautery device. The superior glenohumeral ligament and coracohumeral ligament are also released.
- A full-thickness capsulotomy to a depth of 4 mm within 5–6 mm of the anterior glenoid is performed using an electrocautery and continued from supe-

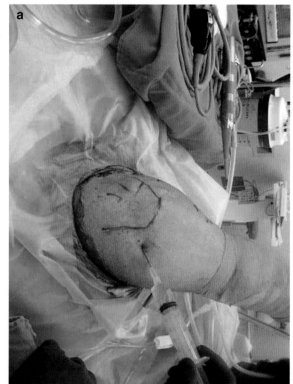

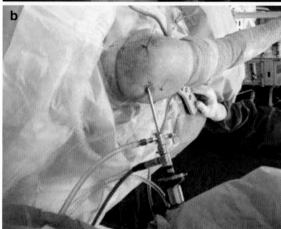

Fig. 8.2 (**a**) Sterile saline solution being injected into the glenohumeral space using an 18-G spinal needle introduced posteriorly. (**b**) Arthroscope introduced through the posterior portal and anterior portal site determined by using a spinal needle

rior to inferior until the interval between the superior border of subscapularis and anterior border of supraspinatus tendon is reached. The anterior release in a right shoulder is performed from the 1

Fig. 8.3 (**a**) Contracted rotator interval. (**b**) Release of rotator interval preceding the anterior capsular release. (**c**) Anterior capsular release using an electrocautery. (**d**) Anterior capsule released

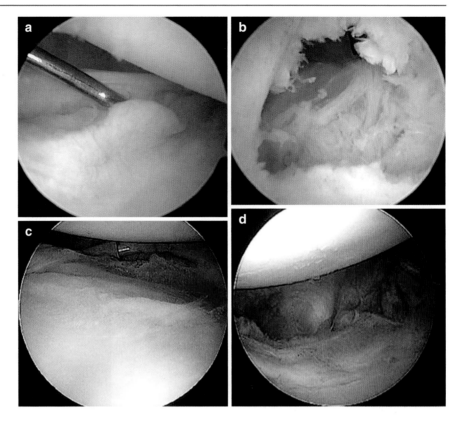

to the 5 o' clock positions and from the 11 to the 7 o' clock positions in a left shoulder (Fig. 8.3a–d).

- As the anterior capsule is divided, rotator interval opens and joint becomes more mobile. The arthroscope is inserted further into the joint anteriorly and inferiorly.
- A soft tissue punch is inserted, placing the blunt jaw exterior to the capsule, and it is divided from anterior to posterior, 5 mm lateral to glenoid labrum. The division is safely carried on to the 5 o' clock position for a right shoulder. Capsulotomy near the glenoid rim in the inferior pouch minimizes the risk of injury to the axillary nerve as the nerve is closest to the capsule at the midpoint of the capsule's glenoid and humeral attachments (Fig. 8.4). The axillary nerve is furthest from the glenoid if the shoulder is placed in abduction and external rotation.
- Alternatively, further release to the axillary pouch can be first addressed from posterior and inferior areas of the capsule.

- At this point, manipulation in forward elevation and abduction-external rotation often releases the inferior pouch.
- If there is still severely limited external rotation after anterior capsular release, surgical release of the superior intraarticular part (25%) of subscapularis tendon can be considered as an option without compromising the musculo-osseous system that resists anterior dislocation.

Posterior Capsule Release

- Posterior capsular release is performed in patients with global loss of motion or persistent limitation of flexion and internal rotation even after anterior release.
- The arthroscope is reversed and placed through the anterosuperior portal (Fig. 8.5) and an electrocautery through the cannula in the posterior portal. The posterior capsule is divided to a depth of 4 mm with

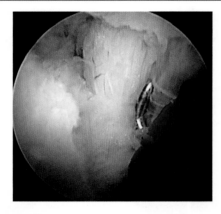

Fig. 8.4 Complete inferior capsular release, axillary nerve with fatty tissue covering, and overlying vasculature along the course of the nerve

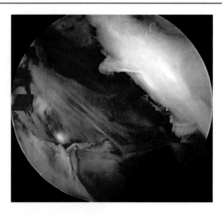

Fig. 8.6 Complete release of posterior capsule, surrounding cuff muscle fibres are visible

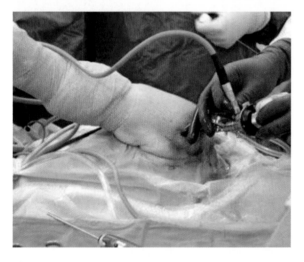

Fig. 8.5 Arthroscope is reversed and introduced through the anterior portal in order to perform posterior capsular release

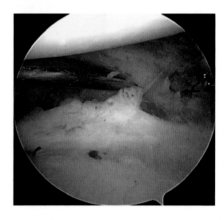

Fig. 8.7 Postreoinferior capsular release using a soft tissue punch

5–6 mm of the posterior glenoid and posterior to the biceps tendon.
- The posterior capsular release is performed from 1 o' clock to 5 o' clock positions in a left shoulder or from 11 o' clock to 7 o' clock positions in a right shoulder.
- The depth of the capsular division is determined when the surgeon sees the cuff muscle fibers (Fig. 8.6).
- Further release of posteroinferior capsule is performed with careful resection using a soft tissue punch and manipulation in abduction-internal rotation (Fig. 8.7).

- After removal of the arthroscope, gentle manipulation of the shoulder is performed routinely and ROM is recorded.

Subacromial Space Evaluation

- All patients should undergo arthroscopic subacromial space evaluation.
- The arthroscope is inserted into the subacromial space through the posterior portal and a 7-mm cannula is introduced through a lateral portal.
- The scar tissue if visible is debrided using the motorized shaver until the rotator cuff is free.

The coracoacromial ligament is released at the base of the coracoid.

- Routine acromioplasty along with capsular release is controversial because of the concern of creating subacromial scarring after acromioplasty.

Postoperative Care

- Rehabilitation program can be a supervised or a home exercise.
- All patients perform home exercise program under supervision on the day of surgery while they are still in hospital.
- The program includes passive forward elevation in supine position, passive external motion with the arm by the side and arm in abduction, assisted passive internal rotation up the back, and assisted cross-body adduction. The patients should continue the exercises for 1 h per day. The patients are not given any sling and encouraged to use the arm in activities of daily living.
- Strengthening and range of motion exercises are begun once the patients have minimal pain, usually around 4–6 weeks after the surgery.

Complications

- Chronic pain and stiffness.
- Instability.
- Articular damage during forceful arthroscopic insertion.
- Manipulation may cause fractures or damage to tendons and ligaments.
- Axillary nerve damage during inferior pouch release.
- Damage to subscapularis tendon.
- Damage to infraspinatus especially during posterior release.

- Dissection medial to the coracoid process places the neurovascular structures such as the musculocutaneous nerve at risk.
- Interscalene block share associated complications (e.g., phrenic or laryngeal nerve block, pneumothorax, toxicity, brachial plexus injury, bronchospasm, or cardiac arrest).

Follow-up

- Patients are seen in the clinic at 1 week for a wound checkup, 2 weeks for removal of sutures, and thereafter at 6 weeks, 3 months, and 6 months.
- If the patient has not achieved satisfactory range of motion after 3–6 months, repeat contracture release may be considered.

Further Reading

Gartsman GM. Shoulder arthroscopy. 1st ed. 2003. p. 143–151; Chap. 6.

Holloway GB, Schenk T, Williams GR, et al. Arthroscopic capsular release for the treatment of refractory postoperative or post-fracture shoulder stiffness. JBJS. 2001;83A(11): 1682–7.

Pollock RG, Duralde XA, Flatow EI, Bigliani LU. Use of arthroscopy in the treatment of resistant frozen shoulder. Clin Orthop Relat Res. 1994;304:30–6.

Warner JJ, Allen A, Marks PH, Wong P. Arthroscopic release of postoperative capsular contracture of the shoulder. JBJS. 1997;79A(8):1151–8.

Warner JJ, Allen A, Marks PH, Wong P. Arthroscopic release of chronic, refractory adhesive capsulitis of the shoulder. JBJS. 1996;78A(12):1808–16.

Snow M, Boutros I, Funk L. Posterior arthroscopic capsular release in frozen shoulder. J Arthros Relat Surg. 2009;25:19–23.

Bunker TD. Arthroscopic capsular release for adhesive capsulitis. Advanced reconstruction of shoulder by Zuckerman. p. 473–479; Chap. 50.

Total Shoulder Arthroplasty in Degenerative Osteoarthritis of the Shoulder

9

George M. Kontakis and Theodoros I. Tosounidis

Indications

Shoulder pain and impaired function due to glenohumeral joint osteoarthritis.

Preoperative Planning

History

- Detailed information regarding the onset and the evolution of his/her symptoms.
- Previous treatments (e.g., joint injections).
- Occupation.
- Socioeconomical status.
- Personality issues (anxiety-motivation-compliance).
- Long medical history, neuromuscular disease as well as previous infection are relative contraindications.

G.M. Kontakis (✉)
Academic Department of Trauma and Orthopaedic Surgery,
School of Medicine, University of Crete,
Heraclion, Crete, Greece
e-mail: gkontaki@yahoo.com

T.I. Tosounidis
Department of Trauma and Orthopaedic Surgery,
Leeds Teaching Hospitals NHS Trust,
Leeds, UK

Clinical Evaluation

- Examine the entire upper limb thoroughly and compare it with the contralateral one.
- Inspect for previous scars and the presence of joint edema.
- Inspect for shoulder muscle atrophy.
- Ask the patient to show tender points or the location of the pain.
- Palpate to define tender points or areas close to the shoulder joint.
- Record the active and the passive range of movements.
- Assess and record any restriction of fixed deformity (external rotation of the arm with the elbow at side that is limited to zero means that a maximum elongation of the subscapularis may be needed; anterior elevation less than 90° means incomplete recovery of this movement after operation).
- Examine the neurovascular status of the upper limb.
- Clear the cervical spine.
- Evaluate the shoulder pain and function using a scoring system (Constant-Murley scale is commonly used in Europe).

Patient's Issues

- Inform the patient about the procedure; analyze the expected benefits and the possible complications.
- Ask for the patient's expectations.

P.V. Giannoudis (ed.), *Practical Procedures in Elective Orthopaedic Surgery*,
DOI 10.1007/978-0-85729-820-1_9, © Springer-Verlag London Limited 2012

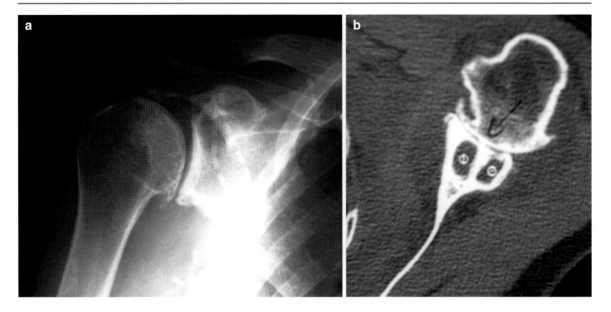

Fig. 9.1 (**a**) Preoperative X-ray. (**b**) CT scan

- Inform the patient in detail about the rehabilitation period, which may be prolonged.
- Assure the patient that this procedure – if uncomplicated – provides sufficient pain relief and improves the overall function.

Imaging

Plain Radiographs

- *True AP shoulder (at the level of the scapula) view shows* (Fig. 9.1a):
  - The acromio-humeral head distance (superior migration of the head when this distance is less than 7 mm means irreparable rotator cuff tear).
  - Narrowing or obliteration of the joint space.
  - The presence of humeral head osteophytes.
  - The possible existence of subchondral cysts.
  - The shape of the glenoid in the scapula level (eccentricity in a vertical direction).
- *Axillary view shows:*
  - The relation of the head with the glenoid.
  - The existence of glenoid osteophytes in the AP direction.
  - The wear of the glenoid bone (centric or eccentric).

CT (Fig. 9.1b)

- Excellent for bone evaluation.
- Detailed information regarding glenoid wear and head eccentricity.
- Evaluation of the glenoid bone stock available for the implantation of the prosthetic glenoid.
- Reveals and classifies fatty degeneration of the rotator cuff.

MRI (Optional)

- In 90% of the patients with degenerative shoulder osteoarthritis, the rotator cuff is intact.
- Assessment of the rotator cuff muscle atrophy or degeneration.

Operative Treatment

Anesthesia

- General anesthesia is used.
- Interscalene block offers good muscle relaxation during the procedure, prolonged postoperative analgesia, and reduced stress response to surgery.

Table and Equipment

- The surgical table should allow patient's positioning in beach-chair position.
- An arm-holder or an arm-supporting Mayo table is utilized.
- Equipment for general shoulder surgery is necessary (special self-retaining retractors, Hohmann retractors, humeral head retractors).
- Complete total shoulder arthroplasty instrumentation.
- Complete series of total shoulder implants (revision stems are included for special situations).
- Strong nonabsorbable sutures (e.g., Ethibond No 5).

Positioning and Surgical Approach

- The patient is positioned in a semi-sitting or beach-chair position with the shoulder (including the scapula) overhanging the lateral edge of the table.
- The head and the thorax are secured to prevent loss of the patient position during the operation and stretching of the cervical nerve roots.
- The arm is rested in a support (a simple arm support fixed laterally on the table facilitating arm position changes during the operation or a sterile dressed Mayo table).
- With a marking pen, draw the acromion, the clavicle, and the coracoid process (Fig. 9.2).
- Skin preparation is carried out using the usual locally applied antiseptics (povidone-iodine or iodine with alcohol). The entire upper extremity is prepped.
- Stockinette is utilized to cover the hand, the forearm, and the lower arm and is secured in place with one or two elastic bandages.
- Sterile adhesive dressing is applied to cover the surgical field including the axilla.
- The exposure is the deltopectoral. The incision is 10–12 cm in length and extends from the lateral clavicle to the upper arm between the deltoid and the lateral margin of the biceps muscle. It passes lateral to the coracoid process. Its length is about 10–12 cm (Fig. 9.3a).
- The cephalic vein is retracted laterally with the deltoid because there are less connecting branches of the vein within the pectoralis major. At the level of the coracoid process, one or two larger vein branches

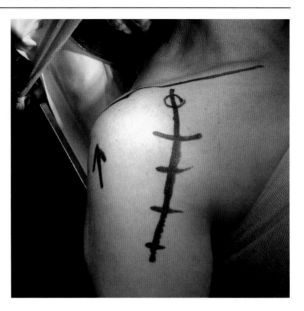

Fig. 9.2 Skin marking

from the pectoralis major the cephalic vein are found, and they are ligated in order to facilitate the exposure. A Hohmann-type retractor is placed over the coracoacromial ligament. The upper 1–2 cm of the pectoralis major insertion is released from the humerus (no need for re-approximation at the end of the procedure).

- The clavipectoral fascia is cut laterally to the conjoined tendon. With the arm in abduction and internal rotation, the deep surface of the deltoid is released from the humerus. Sweeping a finger under the deltoid ensures that the subdeltoid bursa is opened. By placing the arm in flexion and neutral rotation, the conjoined tendon is freed from the subscapularis and retracted medially with a Richardson-type retractor. Subsequently, a self-retaining retractor is utilized (Fig. 9.3b).
- One or two stay sutures are passed through subscapularis in 1 in. distance from its insertion to the lesser tuberosity.
- The anterior circumflex vessels, which are located in the lower edge of the subscapularis, are ligated in 1 cm distance from the humeral head.
- The rotator interval is opened by dull dissection (using the scissor).
- The subscapularis is detached from its insertion at the lesser tuberosity (Fig. 9.3c) preferably with a flake of bone attached to it utilizing a small osteotome.

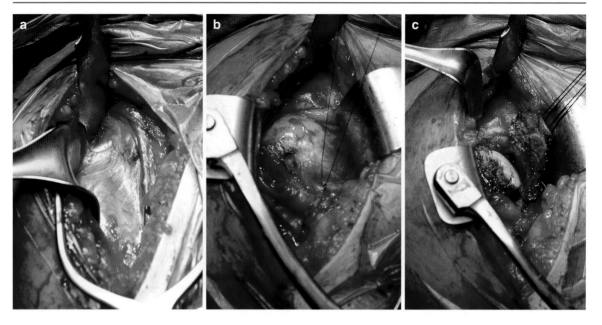

Fig. 9.3 (**a**) Deltopectoral exposure performed. (**b**) Exposure of the humeral head. (**c**) The subscapularis is detached from the lesser tuberosity

- A humeral head retractor (Fukuda) is placed into the joint, retracting the humeral head posteriorly.
- The subscapularis along with the underlying capsule is released superiorly to the base of the coracoid (Fig. 9.4a).
- Then, the anterior part of the joint capsule is divided parallel to the anterior glenoid edge (Fig. 9.4b).
- The inferior capsule is separated from the subscapularis – protecting the axillary nerve – and is cut in an anteroposterior direction (Fig. 9.4c). The subscapularis is now completely released, and its maximal excursion is tested.
- The next step is to disarticulate the humeral head. The arm is placed in extension, slight adduction, and external rotation. Residual release of the inferior joint capsule is performed close to the humeral head.
- Osteophytes are removed from the head with the use of a rongeur and an osteotome to reveal the margin of the anatomical neck exactly (Fig. 9.5).
- Using an oscillating saw, the articular portion of the head is cut parallel to the level of the anatomical head.
- Keep in mind that this articular part of the head is usually thin. To perform a correct head osteotomy, you must cut precisely at the anatomical head level. This ensures the preservation of the rotator cuff insertion and determines the size (diameter) and the

proper orientation of the prosthetic head in relation to the transepicondylar axis (retroversion).
- The humeral canal is opened with an awl. The entry point is just behind the upper part of the bicipital groove. The canal is prepared initially by the use of cylindrical reamers in order to determine its diameter (Fig. 9.6a).
- The humeral-head-metaphyseal angle is measured, and the site where the lateral fin of the prosthesis fits is marked posteriorly. This allows for the implantation of the prosthesis with the proper retroversion.
- The humeral canal is then prepared by the use of the appropriate rasps (Fig. 9.6b).
- A trial prosthesis is implanted, and the offsets for the permanent prosthesis are assessed (Figs. 9.6c, d).
- The trial prosthesis is removed, and a protective non-implantable stem is inserted.
- A pronged retractor is placed to the anterior neck of the glenoid, and a Fukuda retractor is inserted. The glenoid is exposed for preparation.
- The labrum is incised circumferentially, and a careful soft tissue release posteriorly allows for the maximum field to be gained.
- Osteophytes are removed with a thin osteotome.
- The center of the glenoid is determined, a central hole is opened (Fig. 9.7a), and reaming is performed

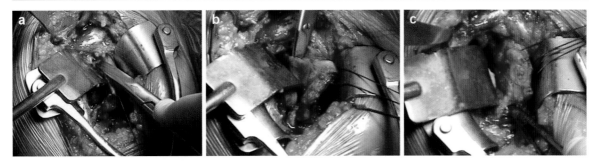

Fig. 9.4 (**a–c**) The steps of the capsular exposure and subscapularis release

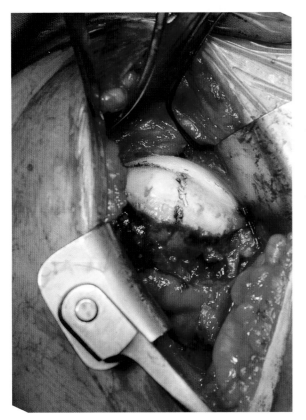

Fig. 9.5 The anatomic humeral neck is exposed following osteophyte removal

follows. A reduction is performed, and the adequacy of the soft tissue balance is tested. With the head reduced and facing to the glenoid, an anteroposterior force is applied. Normally, the head should be subluxed posteriorly less than half of its diameter and must be reduced automatically when the force is removed.

- If the head is permanently subluxed or dislocated posteriorly, a posterior capsulorrhaphy (from an anterior to posterior direction) should be performed after implantation of the permanent prosthesis.
- A cemented prosthetic glenoid is inserted first (Fig. 9.8a, b).
- Wait for cement consolidation (applying force to the prosthetic glenoid with a proper impactor).
- Three to four strong nonabsorbable sutures are passed through the bone, laterally to the bicipital groove for the final site of the re-opposition of the subscapularis (Fig. 9.9).
- After the implantation of the cemented humeral component (Fig. 9.10), and cement consolidation, reduction of the joint is performed. The subscapularis is sutured back to the upper humeral metaphysis, and the rotator interval is closed.
- The range of motion is assessed and recorded with the arm close to the side, and the rotation is additionally evaluated in 90° abduction.

(Fig. 9.7b). Depending on the type of the glenoid implant (keeled or with pegs), the surface of the glenoid is prepared accordingly.
- Bear in mind that for a correct glenoid preparation, you must be able to work easily with straight instruments.
- Finishing the configuration of the glenoid bed (Fig. 9.7c), a trial glenoid component is put in place, and the humeral head trial prosthesis placement

Closure

- A suction drain is placed.
- The deltopectoral interval is closed with loose sutures.
- The fascia is closed with the use of interrupted sutures.
- Skin closure is performed typically with sutures or staples.

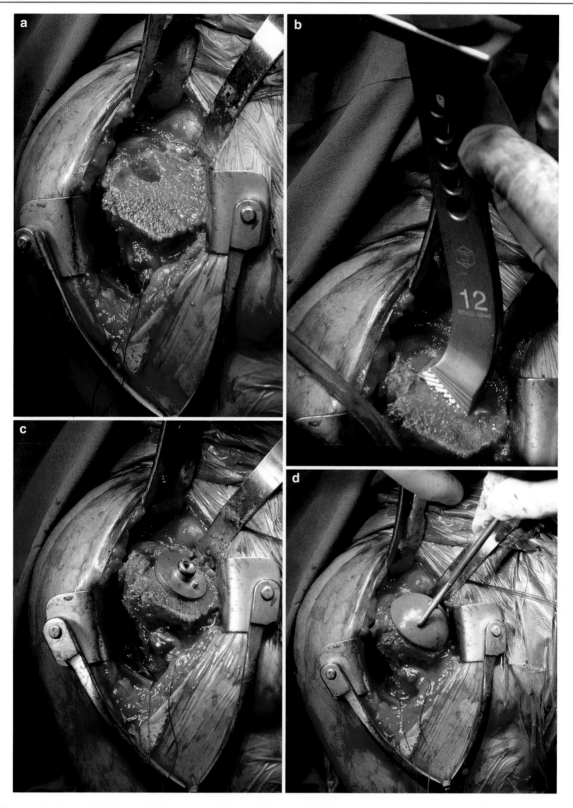

Fig. 9.6 (**a**) The canal is initially prepared with specific reamers. (**b**) The humeral canal is prepared with the use of appropriate rasps. (**c**) The humeral trial prosthesis is inserted. (**d**) The appropriate size of a trial humeral head is connected with the humeral stem

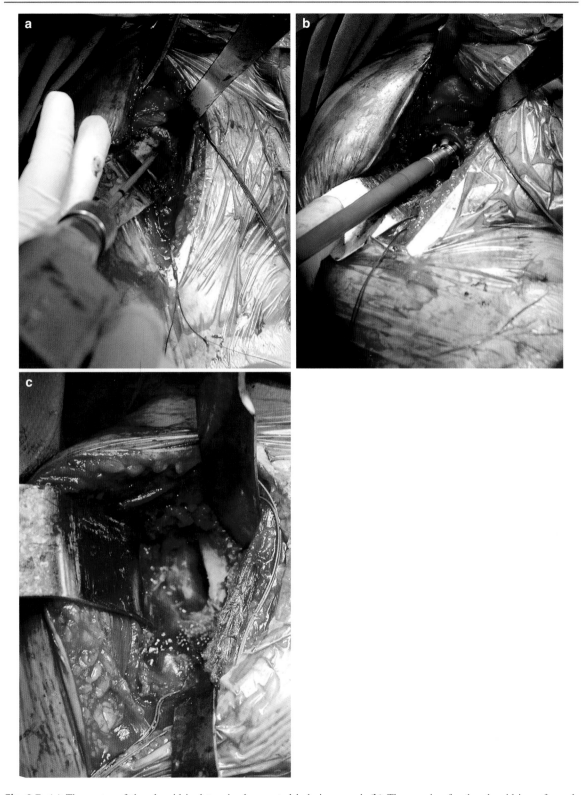

Fig. 9.7 (**a**) The center of the glenoid is determined, a central hole is opened. (**b**) The reaming for the glenoid is performed. (**c**) Finalization of the glenoid

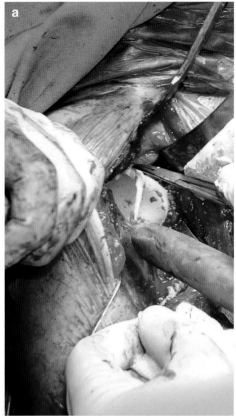

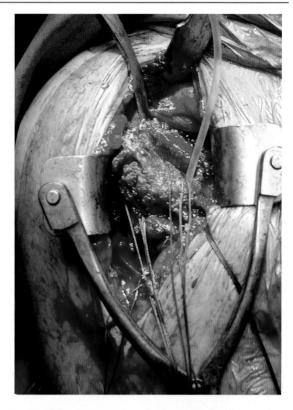

Fig. 9.9 Three to four strong nonabsorbable sutures are passed through the bone, laterally to the bicipital groove for the final site of the re-opposition of the subscapularis

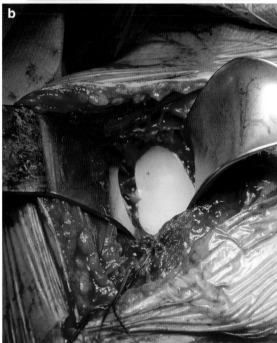

Fig. 9.8 (**a**) A cemented prosthetic glenoid is inserted. (**b**) The prosthesis (*closer view*)

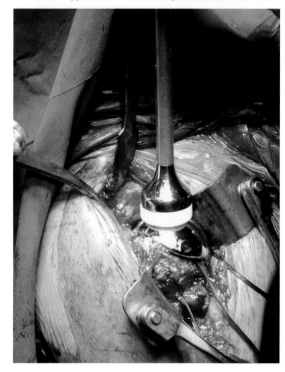

Fig. 9.10 The implantation of the humeral component is performed

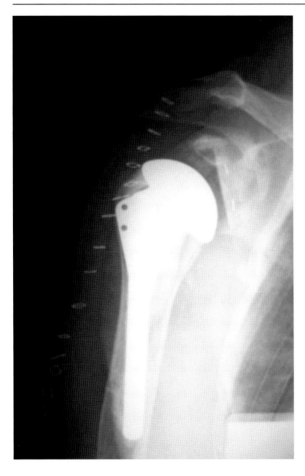

Fig. 9.11   Postoperative X-ray

Postoperative Rehabilitation and Follow-up

- Wrist, elbow, and pendulum exercises for the shoulder are encouraged from the first postoperative day. A postoperative X-ray is required (Fig. 9.11).

- The patient is instructed to perform passive and assisted active shoulder flexion movements. As pain subsides, the range of the movements is increased. External rotation beyond 10° is avoided during the first 3 weeks.
- Isometric shoulder muscle strengthening is permitted (except from strengthening of the internal rotators in order to protect subscapularis tendon healing).
- Stretching exercises – for achievement of range of motion – and active shoulder exercises are more intense after 6 weeks post-surgery.
- The physiotherapy program may be continued during the first 6 months.
- Follow-up appointments are at 3 and 6 weeks, at 3 and 6 months, and at 1 year.

Further Reading

Neer CS2nd. Articular replacement for the humeral head. J Bone Joint Surg Am. 1955;37-A:215–28.

Rodosky MW, Bigliani LU. Indications for glenoid resurfacing in shoulder arthroplasty. J Shoulder Elbow Surg. 1996; 5:231–48.

Cofield RH. Total shoulder arthroplasty with the Neer prosthesis. J Bone Joint Surg Am. 1984;66:899–906.

Godeneche A, Boileau P, Favard L, Le Huec JC, Levigne C, Nove-Josserand L, et al. Prosthetic replacement in the treatment of osteoarthritis of the shoulder: early results of 268 cases. J Shoulder Elbow Surg. 2002;11:11–8.

Boileau P, Avidor C, Krishnan SG, Walch G, Kempf JF, Mole D. Cemented polyethylene versus uncemented metal-backed glenoid components in total shoulder arthroplasty: a prospective, double-blind, randomized study. J Shoulder Elbow Surg. 2002;11:351–9.

Boileau P, Walch G. Technique of glenoid resurfacing in shoulder arthroplasty. In: Boileau P, Walch G, editors. Shoulder arthroplasty. Berlin: Springer; 1999. p. 147–62.

Part II

Upper Extremity: Humerus – Elbow

Nonunions of the Humeral Shaft: Open Reduction Plate Fixation and Autologous Bone Graft Augmentation

10

Nikolaos K. Kanakaris, Fragkiskos N. Xypnitos, and Peter V. Giannoudis

Introduction

- The incidence of humeral nonunions ranges from 2% to 10% (literature of initial nonoperative treatment of humeral fractures) to 12–15% (literature of initial operative treatment of humeral fractures).
- Associated risk factors are:
  - The severity of the initial injury
  - Open fractures
  - Bone loss
  - Transverse fracture patterns
  - Distraction at the fracture site
  - Soft tissue interposition
  - Infection
  - Inadequate immobilization
  - Obesity or large body habitus
  - Osteoporosis
  - Alcoholism
  - Smoking
  - Malnutrition
  - Noncompliance to management plan

N.K. Kanakaris (✉)
Department of Trauma and Orthopaedic Surgery,
Leeds Teaching Hospitals NHS Trust,
Leeds, UK
e-mail: nikolaoskanakaris@yahoo.co.uk

F.N. Xypnitos
Department of Trauma and Orthopaedics,
Leeds Teaching Hospitals NHS Trust,
Leeds, UK

P.V. Giannoudis
Academic Department of Trauma and Orthopaedic Surgery,
School of Medicine, University of Leeds,
Leeds, UK

- The vast majority of humeral nonunions require operative management to relieve instability, pain, and disability of the extremity.
- Their treatment differs from that of acute fractures as it often requires intrafocal debridement of the nonunion site, and the operation is often complicated by the presence of hardware (plate or nail), bone loss, or infection.
- Nonunion can be classified as hypertrophic or oligo/atrophic, septic or non-septic, and with or without the presence of hardware. It is imperative that all such cases are carefully assessed and the management plan carefully set by an experienced, in such cases, orthopedic team.

Preoperative Planning

Clinical Assessment

- The complete medical history of the patient and of the sequel of events since the initial injury should be carefully reviewed, especially for symptoms that could be associated with the presence of a current or previous local infection.
- Identify and address, as many as possible, associated predisposing factors (i.e., nutrition supplements, decrease smoking, mechanical stability, biologic enhancement-grafting, etc.).
- Physical examination of the involved extremity should identify the presence of sinuses (active or not), focal or generalized inflammation, axillary lymphadenopathy, neurovascular status, and functional level of adjacent joints.

P.V. Giannoudis (ed.), *Practical Procedures in Elective Orthopaedic Surgery*,
DOI 10.1007/978-0-85729-820-1_10, © Springer-Verlag London Limited 2012

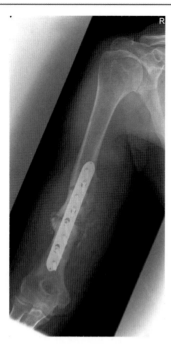

Fig. 10.1 X-ray demonstrating a humeral nonunion with a plate inserted posteriorly

- Basic blood tests should include full blood count CRP and ESR levels that can be indicative of the presence of sepsis. Unexplained anemia, serum hypoalbuminemia, or a cachectic general appearance may indicate nutritional deficiencies that need to be addressed before surgery.

Radiological Assessment

- Two level plain X-rays of the nonunion site and the adjacent joints remain the gold standard imaging investigations (Fig. 10.1).
- CT scan is useful for preoperative planning of the nonunion debridement, the identification of sequestrum, and areas of partial bone healing that will need to be osteotomized.
- Bone scintigraphy with gallium-67 can be useful whereas septic environment is suspected. Guided aspiration of the nonunion site and microbiologic examination of the aspirate may also be considered in the pre-operative assessment phase.

Timing of Surgery

- The diagnosis of a potential humeral shaft nonunion should be set once bone healing is radiologically

inadequate after the 16th week post-injury and the extremity symptomatic and painful in plain activities.
- In general, the prolongation of the patient's incapacity should be avoided, and early intervention should precede the establishment of a complete nonunion (after the 36th week post-injury) in those patients that are closely followed-up and do not have any other comorbidities that contradict surgery.

Operative Procedure

Anesthesia

- General anesthesia is usually preferable to allow for the procedure at the nonunion site as well as for bone graft harvesting from the pelvis.
- Local anesthetic may also be used at the surgical incision of the humerus as well as to that of the iliac crest, offering temporary pain relief.
- Administration of prophylactic antibiotics as per hospital protocol (e.g., single dose of iv 1.5 g Cefuroxime, 1.2 g Co-amoxiclav, or 400 mg Teicoplanin), or it is held before the acquisition of intraoperative cultures, in suspected infection.

Table and Equipment

- Large fragment (4.5 mm) LC-DCP or LCP plating set
- Osteotomes set (±) autograft set
- Standard osteosynthesis set as per local hospital protocol
- Radiolucent table (±) Mayo table (depending of the position of the patient at the table and the chosen approach)
- Fluoroscopy

Table Setup

- The instrumentation is set up on the side of the operation.
- The image intensifier comes from the ipsilateral side when needed.
- The image intensified screen should be at contralateral side.

Fig. 10.2 A typical beach-chair position. In the majority of the cases, it is advised to leave the elbow joint uncovered

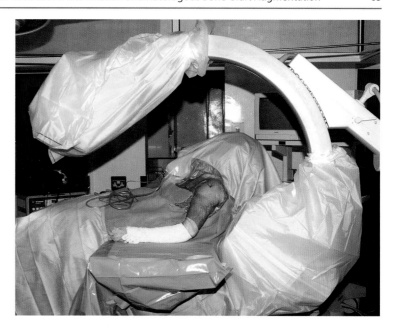

- Position the table diagonally across the operating square field covered by the laminar flow.

Patient Positioning

- This will be dictated by the chosen approach to the nonunion site. Associated is also the presence of any previous operation scars. Usually the same approach to that of the primary ORIF is selected.
- If nonoperative treatment or a nailing was initially performed, then for diaphyseal nonunions, a posterior approach is usually preferred with the patient in a lateral decubitus position. The upper extremity is supported by a padded post as well as the patient's body supported with the appropriate padded posts. In-between the legs, a pillow may be useful, as well as padding of the lower leg at the areas of the ankle and the fibular head.
- If the nonunion site is extending proximally to the upper one-third of the shaft, or if the original fixation was served by an extended anterolateral approach, then the patient is positioned either supine or in the beach-chair position (Fig. 10.2), with the arm resting on a draped Mayo table.
- Prior to skin prepping and draping, the surgeon must confirm that good quality fluoroscopic images can be obtained.

Draping and Surgical Exposure

- Prepare the skin of the whole arm including the shoulder, using usual antiseptic solutions (aqueous or alcoholic povidone-iodine or chlorhexidine).
- Use isolation drapes for the armpit.
- The arm is draped free using U-drapes over the side of the table with the elbow flexed (lateral decubitus position – posterior approach).
- The arm and forearm are prepped and draped with a stockinet and crepe bandage.

Anterolateral Approach

- The incision follows a line extending distally from the interval between the biceps and the brachioradialis and the wrist extensors to the deltopectoral interval proximally, following the lateral edge of biceps (Fig. 10.3a, b).
- Incise the fascia carefully between biceps/brachilis and the mobile wad and extend proximally (Fig. 10.3c).
- Be aware of the lateral cutaneous nerve crossing distally. The radial nerve which is deeper should be identified and protected. Also, proximally, indentify the cephalic vein in the deltopectoral interval.
- Retract the biceps and brachialis medially and the mobile wad laterally in order to identify the radial

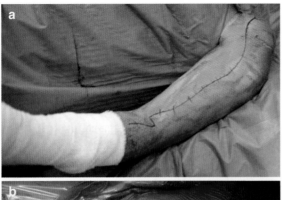

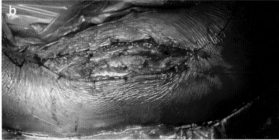

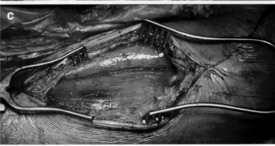

Fig. 10.3 (**a**) Skin marking and draping for the anterolateral approach. (**b**) The lateral edge of the biceps is identified. (**c**) Incise the fascia between biceps/brachialis and the mobile wad

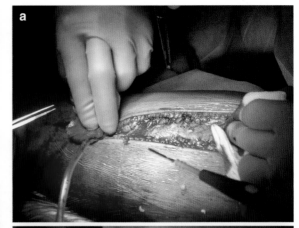

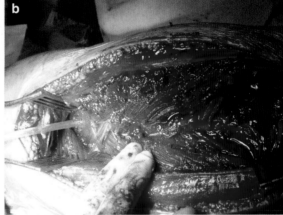

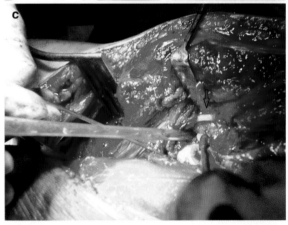

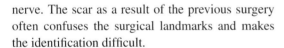

Fig. 10.4 (**a**) Incised skin and subcutaneous fat. (**b**) The two part (heads) of the triceps are retracted medially and laterally. (**c**) The radial nerve (*arrow* is indentified) and protected

nerve. The scar as a result of the previous surgery often confuses the surgical landmarks and makes the identification difficult.

- Mobilize the radial nerve, as needed, to access the bone. Follow the nerve to the point where it passes through the lateral intermuscular septum.
- It is advisable to preserve muscular attachments, avoiding further devascularization of the bone.

Posterior Approach

- Skin landmarks: tip of the olecranon, posterior edge of the acromion, and medial and lateral epicondyles. Midline posterior marking: from the level of the distal border of the deltoid to the tip of the olecranon.
- Incise in the skin, subcutaneous fat, and fascia (Fig. 10.4a).

- Identify the tendon and each one of triceps' superficial heads (lateral and long head).
- Start dissecting proximally between the two superficial heads and continue distally at the same direction by sharp dissection of the tendon (Fig. 10.4b).
- Identify and preserve the inferior lateral cutaneous brachial nerve (branch of the radial nerve).
- Retract the long and lateral heads of the triceps from each other and identify carefully the radial nerve (Fig. 10.4c) and the profunda branchial artery in the spiral groove, covered by the medial head of the triceps. In the case of nonunions, these steps should be done cautiously due to the scar tissue and the potential displacement of these elements due to previous operations, scars, and callus. They may be partially or fully covered – entrapped within the callus and scar tissue. Careful dissection, mobilization from distal to proximal, tagging with a rubber sling, and continuous protection are essential steps during this procedure. The lateral intermuscular septum usually is divided for further mobilization of the radial nerve and distal exposure.
- The medial head is dissected sharply from the periosteum in a medial to lateral direction, and the nonunion site should be fully and circumferentially exposed.

Nonunion Debridement

- The nonunion site is fully exposed and debrided to healthy bleeding, viable bone. All scar tissue, soft callus, and synovial tissue (in the true pseudarthrosis cases) must be resected. Osteotomes, curettes, and rongeurs are used for that purpose.
- Multiple specimens are obtained with different forceps and sent in different pots for gram stain and full microbiology analysis and culture.
- All previous metalwork is removed, including broken implants.
- The intramedullary canal is also opened via 3.5- and 4.5-mm drill bits and hand reamers, establishing potentially an endosteal source of osteoprogenitor cells to the nonunion level.
- Oblique shortening osteotomies may be necessary to allow for correction of any deformity and to achieve apposition of the bone ends. Loss of length of 3–4 cm for the humeral diaphysis appears to have no particular effect to the function of the adjacent joints and the muscle strength of the elbow.
- Such osteotomies are best done with a saw blade, which need to be cooled at the time with irrigation of saline, while the radial nerve is gently protected.
- By creating two oblique contact areas of the main fragments, a lag screw can also be placed to facilitate compression and increase the stability of the fixation.

Late Evidence of Infection

- Preoperative thorough clinical, radiological, and laboratory evaluation should always attempt to clarify the presence or absence of local sepsis. The treatment algorithm of septic nonunions differs significantly and may lead to a staged approach instead of the one-stage fixation and grafting.
- In those cases where, besides all negative preoperative results, after exposure of the nonunion site there is macroscopic evidence of sepsis (pus around the old fixation and non-healing humeral shaft fracture), or the urgent gram stain of the intraoperative samples is positive, the operative-grafting plan should be altered.
- In overall healthy patients, compression plate fixation should continue as originally planned, avoiding however the autologous bone-grafting stage. Antibiotic-impregnated calcium sulfate (osteoconductive agent as well as delivery vehicle of local antibiotics) or antibiotic-impregnated methylmethacrylate cement beads may be inserted at the infected nonunion site.
- In the presence of gross infection (extremely rare in those cases where, preoperatively all investigations were proven negative) or if the host suffers from serious comorbidities (diabetes, immunosuppression, cancer, etc.), the nonunion site should be temporarily stabilized with an external fixator, and a staged approach should follow with serial debridement until definitive fixation. The application of a circular fixator may also offer the means of definitive fixation especially in compromised patients or/and multiresistant microorganisms.

Grafting

- Especially for oligo/atrophic nonunions, the element of biological enhancement of the nonunion site with bone graft is of paramount importance.

- In the literature, there are reports of using, instead of the gold standard of iliac crest autologous cancellous bone graft, other materials (i.e., BMPs, demineralized bone matrix, fibular allograft, or composite grafts). Besides the donor-site morbidity and the quantity restriction of autograft, it remains the method used at the vast majority of cases.
- Please see clear description at the chapter of "Bone Graft Harvesting" in the present book. All necessary precautions and considerations should be taken while positioning and draping the patient, so that easy access to the anterior iliac crest is feasible at the time of the nonunion operation.

Implant and Graft Positioning

- Compression osteosynthesis with the use of a large fragment 4.5-mm LC-DCP or LCP plate with optimally the addition of a 4.5-mm interfragmentary lag screw is performed laterally or anterolaterally (to the tension side of the humerus).
- The length of the plate must allow at least four screws (eight cortices) to be used above and below the nonunion level, or three screws (six cortices) if a lag screw has been also applied.
- Prebending and overcontouring of the plate may be necessary to produce compression to the far cortex of the humeral shaft.
- The bone graft is applied in the medullary canal, at the nonunion site prior to plate fixation, and around the nonunion site circumferentially after the plate fixation.
- Reduction and application of the implants must be done mostly by direct reduction techniques in the most possible atraumatic way in order to preserve the vascularity of the surrounding soft tissues.
- The screws should be inserted in an offset pattern and different planes than parallel to reduce the risk of fatigue fractures through rotational load and avoid fissuring or splitting of the diaphysis.
- Protect the radial nerve in all stages, and make sure it is loosely mobilized and not entrapped or stretched at the edges of the plate.
- Implant position and nonunion reduction and alignment are confirmed using fluoroscopic imaging.

Closure and Dressings

- Irrigation of the wound and cautious hemostasis.
- Closure in layers preferably with interrupted sutures using number 1 vicryl for the fascia, 2.0 vicryl for the subcutaneous fat, and interrupted matrix 2.0 nylon sutures for the skin closure.
- Dressings are applied as well as wool bandage starting from distally below the wrist and extending above the elbow close to the axilla.
- A long-arm back slab with the elbow in 90° of flexion is applied as well as collar and cuff or a Bradford sling for overnight elevation.

Postoperative Care and Rehabilitation

- Neurovascular status is meticulously checked and documented at the recovery room.
- Standard laboratory tests as per hospital protocol are required at the first postop day.
- Radiographs are taken usually during the first 48 h (Fig. 10.5).
- A wound check and assessment of its healing is usually necessary before patient's discharge, usually the second postoperative day.
- A split back slab (Jig saw plaster) can be applied for the first 2 weeks, leaving the wrist usually free, and this can stay for comfort and to allow wound inspection and the initial swelling to settle.
- Patients are placed in a sling, which can be removed to permit active exercises of the shoulder and elbow. Gentle pendulum exercises of the shoulder and range of motion of the elbow can be started at 2 weeks postoperatively together with skin suture removal.
- After the 4th to 6th week, strengthening and passive range of motion exercises may follow.

Outpatient Follow-up

- Follow-up X-rays are useful at the 2nd month from surgery, unless there is clinical suspicion of infection, implant failure, or persistent pain.

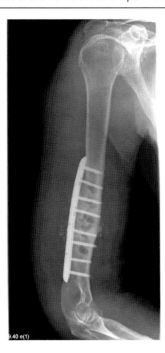

Fig. 10.5 Postoperative X-rays of the patient with the posterior approach and the exchange platting (from Fig. 10.1)

- The average time to union varies significantly depending on biological and mechanical parameters, ranging from 3 to 9 months.
- Standard radiological criteria (callus formation bridging three out of four cortices) are used for this period of assessment.

Complications

- Neurovascular injury.
- Infection.
- Persistent nonunion.
- Decreased arm function due to shortening of the humerus and subsequently of the lever arm of the arm muscles.
- Persistent joint stiffness (elbow or shoulder).
- Algodystrophy.

Further Reading

Rubel IF, Kloen P, Campbell D, et al. Open reduction and internal fixation of humeral nonunions: a biomechanical and clinical study. J Bone Joint Surg Am. 2002;84-A:1315–22.

Pugh DM, McKee MD. Advances in the management of humeral nonunion. J Am Acad Orthop Surg. 2003;11:48–59.

Hierholzer C, Sama D, Toro JB, et al. Plate fixation of ununited humeral shaft fractures: effect of type of bone graft on healing. J Bone Joint Surg Am. 2006;88:1442–7.

Kanakaris NK, Giannoudis PV. The health economics of the treatment of long-bone non-unions. Injury. 2007;38 Suppl 2:S77–84.

Brennan ML, Taitsman LA, Barei DP, et al. Shortening osteotomy and compression plating for atrophic humeral nonunions: surgical technique. J Orthop Trauma. 2008;22:643–7.

Giannoudis PV, Kanakaris NK, Dimitriou R, et al. The synergistic effect of autograft and BMP-7 in the treatment of atrophic nonunions. Clin Orthop Relat Res. 2009;467:3239–48.

Repair of the Ruptured Distal Biceps Tendon

David Limb

Indications

- Rupture of the distal biceps tendon in a patient who wishes to undergo repair after consideration of the risks and rewards.
- Repair is more likely to result in normal strength but will keep the individual off of work that involves heavy lifting and contact sport for at least 3 months.
- Without repair, flexion strength will return close to normal due to brachialis hypertrophy, but there is a more significant deficit in supination strength.

Preoperative Planning

Clinical Assessment

- The diagnosis can usually be confidently made on clinical observation.
- The history usually involves biceps overload, usually with an eccentric contraction (e.g., trying to keep hold of a falling weight that is too heavy to control) and often with a "snap" felt by the patient.
- There is flattening of the arm above the cubital fossa due to retraction of the belly of biceps.

D. Limb
Leeds General Infirmary,
Leeds, UK
e-mail: d.limb@leeds.ac.uk

Radiological Assessment

- Radiographs are noncontributory.
- If confirmation of the clinical diagnosis is required, this can be achieved with ultrasound examination.

Operative Technique

Anesthesia

- General anesthesia is induced and prophylactic antibiotics are administered before application of an above-elbow tourniquet.
- Although in theory the tourniquet could trap the biceps belly that has retracted, in practice there is not usually any problem restoring biceps length by gentle traction on the tendon stump.

Positioning and Equipment

- The patient is positioned supine with the arm on a side table.
- Whereas many operations on a side table are most conveniently carried out with the surgeon seated on the axillary side of the table, access for distal biceps repair is most easily achieved from the head end of the side table.
- A basic tray contains all the equipment needed for the approach and retrieval of the tendon. Specialist equipment depends on the needs of the particular technique.

P.V. Giannoudis (ed.), *Practical Procedures in Elective Orthopaedic Surgery*,
DOI 10.1007/978-0-85729-820-1_11, © Springer-Verlag London Limited 2012

- Recently, good results have been described by approaching entirely through the cubital fossa, fixing the tendon with suture anchors or a tenodesis screw but this approach is associated with a higher risk of neurological injury. This chapter describes the traditional two incision technique, which employs a smaller cubital approach and a suture repair.

Surgical Approach

- A 2-cm incision is made in the center of the elbow flexion crease (Fig. 11.1). Care is taken to preserve the cubital vein and the medial cutaneous nerve of the forearm, which can cross this incision. The fat layer is opened by blunt dissection to reach the fascia that is often disrupted where the lacertus fibrosus has been torn.

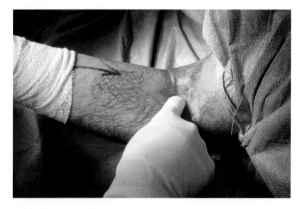

Fig. 11.1 Localizing for the cubital incision by palpating the hollow medial to the mobile wad

- The index finger is inserted and the distal biceps tendon is palpated proximally and retrieved through the wound. The avulsed stump is often expanded (Fig. 11.2a) and should be trimmed to a constant diameter before inserting two No. 2 nonabsorbable sutures (e.g., Ethibond) at right angles as a weave (Fig. 11.2b). The two ends of each suture are left long, so that the stump has four lengths of projecting suture material.
- The index finger can be slid down the track of the avulsed tendon to palpate the bicipital tuberosity of the radius, from which the tendon has avulsed.
- A long, curved clip is passed down to the tuberosity and is slid around the interosseous border of the radius with the tip of the curve directed towards the radius.
- After passing the ulnar side of the radius, the clip is pushed through muscle to tent the skin. A 2.5–3 cm incision is made and centered on the clip, and the clip is withdrawn.
- Through this incision, the muscle is split in the line of its fibers to expose the radius – full pronation brings the bicipital tuberosity into the base of the wound (Fig. 11.3a).

Surgical Procedure

- A large burr is used to open the bicipital tuberosity, creating an opening as large as the diameter of the biceps tendon stump (Fig. 11.3b). The forearm is then supinated to a neutral position and three 2-mm

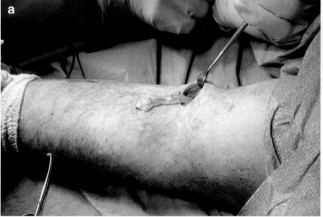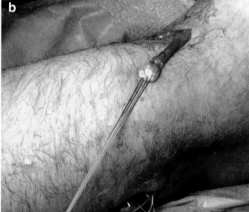

Fig. 11.2 (**a**) The stump of the avulsed biceps tendon. (**b**) Two sutures are woven into the distal stump and a long curved clip is passed around the border of the radius with its curve facing away from the ulna. It is pushed to tent the skin and localize the radial incision

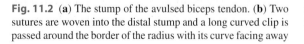

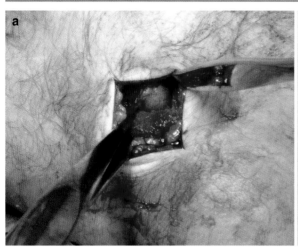 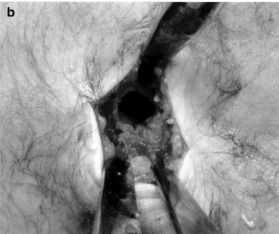

Fig. 11.3 (**a**) The bare tuberosity from which the biceps insertion has been avulsed. (**b**) A hole has been burred into the radial tuberosity to accept the biceps tendon

drill holes are made through the radius to enter the cavity created by the burr above.

- Bone debris is washed out to reduce the risk of heterotopic bone formation and cross union.
- The four suture ends projecting from the biceps stump are held in the tip of the curved clip, which is again passed through from the cubital incision to the radial incision. The sutures are pulled through to draw the biceps tendon to the radius.
- The four suture ends are passed into the cavity created in the bicipital tuberosity and out through the three drill holes. Clearly this will mean that two of the sutures have to pass through one of the holes. This pair should include one strand from each of the two sutures woven into biceps.
- With the forearm supinated, the four suture ends are pulled to draw the biceps stump into the tuberosity. Satisfactory seating can be checked by pronation whilst maintaining tension on the sutures – this brings the biceps tendon into view as it enters the cavity in the tuberosity.
- When satisfied that the biceps is properly seated, the two pairs of sutures are tied over bone bridges and the integrity of the biceps repair is checked through the anterior wound (Fig. 11.4). Full range of pronation and supination is checked before closure.
- Fat is closed with an absorbable suture and skin, with an absorbable subcuticular suture (Fig. 11.5a, b).
- An above-elbow backslab is applied with the forearm in a neutral position, such that the repaired tendon is between radius and ulna. Immobilization in supination may result in a significant problem attempting to regain pronation afterwards.

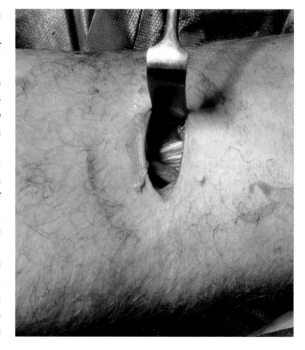

Fig. 11.4   The completed repair

Postoperative Care and Rehabilitation

- After 2–3 weeks, the plaster backslab is replaced by a hinged brace with elastic outriggers.
- A free range of movement is allowed, but firm elastic is connected to eyelets created at the proximal end of the upper arm component and distal end of the forearm component.

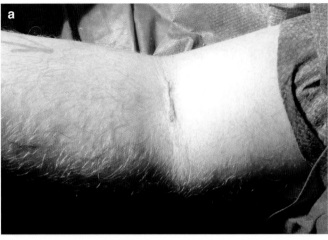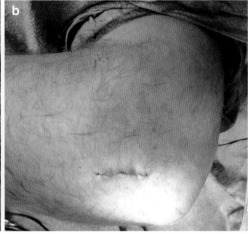

Fig. 11.5 (a) The cubital incision after closure. (b) The radial incision closed

- Thus, extension requires muscular force to stretch the elastic outrigger, but flexion is passive as the elastic returns to its original length.
- The brace is removed 6 weeks after surgery, and active strengthening is commenced. Full effort lifting and unprotected sport is avoided until the 6 month mark.

Complications

- Heterotopic ossification, particularly into the insertion of the tendon into the radius, which can block rotation. This can occur with suture anchor methods just as it can occur with the two-incision technique historically cross union has been reported with the 2 incision technique but this is very rare using the modified technique described above.
- Nerve injury. Care has to be taken to stick to the smoothly walled track of the biceps tendon when dissecting or palpating down to identify the bicipital tuberosity.
- Elbow stiffness, particularly rotation. Prolonged casting should be avoided and cast bracing instituted to protect the repair whilst allowing a full range of flexion and extension.
- Re-rupture. Fortunately very rare in all reported studies, though publication bias means that smaller series with complication rates a little higher than seen in larger series are unlikely to be published.

Results

- After distal biceps tendon repair, a return to full strength is expected, though the biceps does tend to

waste when in a dynamic brace and full strength is not generally achieved for approximately 6 months.
- Cosmetically, the contour of the biceps is expected to return to normal.

Follow-up

- A 3-week appointment for clinical assessment is suggested. Following that, a 3- and 6-month appointment should be given.
- I didn't say this and this may vary between countries. In the UK it is the patients responsibility to ensure they are safe to control the vehicle and it is not up to the surgeon to say that driving is allowed after any particular time for a given procedure

Further Reading

Johnson TS, Johnson DC, Shindle MK, et al. One- versus two-incision technique for distal biceps tendon repair. HSS J. 2008;4(2):117–22; Epub 2008 Aug 22.

Hamer MJ, Caputo AE. Operative treatment of chronic distal biceps tendon ruptures. Sports Med Arthrosc. 2008;16(3):143–7.

Mazzocca AD, Spang JT, Arciero RA. Distal biceps rupture. Orthop Clin North Am. 2008;39(2):237–49.

Henry J, Feinblatt J, Kaeding CC, et al. Biomechanical analysis of distal biceps tendon repair methods. Am J Sports Med. 2007;35(11):1950–4.

Sotereanos DG, Pierce TD, Varitimidis SE. A simplified method for repair of distal biceps tendon ruptures. J Shoulder Elbow Surg. 2000;9(3):227–33.

Subcutaneous Ulnar Nerve Transposition

12

Robert Farnell

Indications

- Cubital tunnel syndrome that has not responded to nonoperative treatment.

Contraindications

- Active infection.
- CRPS.

Preoperative Planning

Clinical Assessment

- Ensure the cubital tunnel syndrome remains symptomatic.
- Review nerve conduction studies where available.

Radiological Assessment

- X-rays are not necessary unless cubitus valgus or elbow osteoarthritis is considered to be an etiological factor.

R. Farnell
Department of Trauma and Orthopaedic Surgery,
Leeds Teaching Hospitals NHS Trust,
Leeds, UK
e-mail: robert.farnell@leedsth.nhs.uk

Preoperative Consent

- Fully explain the procedure and that there will be a permanent visible scar.
- Discuss the postoperative risks including wound infection, elbow stiffness, bleeding, and injury to the ulnar or medial antebrachial cutaneous nerves (usually results in temporary numbness or paresthesia, but it may be permanent with hypersensitivity).
- Mark the limb.

Operative Treatment

Anesthesia

- General or regional anesthesia (brachial plexus block).

Equipment

- Standard hand surgical equipment tray.
- Bipolar diathermy.

Patient Positioning

- Patient supine with the arm lying on an arm table which is attached to the operating table.
- Fit a high arm pneumatic tourniquet. It is important to ensure this is as near to the axilla as possible.

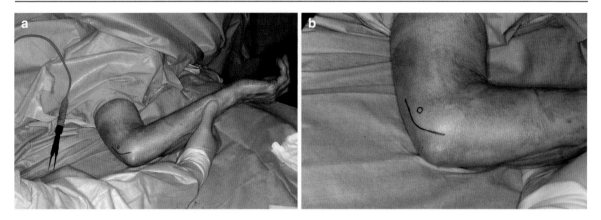

Fig. 12.1 (**a**) Preparation of the arm with a high pneumatic tourniquet, an arm table, and upper extremity drape. Note that the tourniquet has been placed as proximal as possible. (**b**) Skin marking showing the medial epicondyle and skin incision site

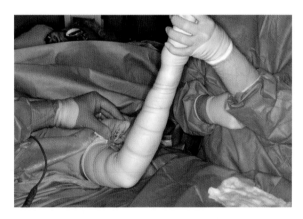

Fig. 12.2 Exsanguination of arm with a sterile Esmarch bandage

Draping and Surgical Approach

- Prepare the skin of the hand, forearm, and upper arm to the level of the tourniquet using your usual antiseptic solutions (e.g., aqueous povidone-iodine).
- Use an upper extremity exclusion drape which also covers the arm table (Fig. 12.1a). Gently externally rotate the arm and put an upturned bowl beneath the elbow. Be careful not to forcibly externally rotate the shoulder to prevent injury.
- Draw your skin incision with a skin marking pen, which is a curved incision posterior to the medial epicondyle (Fig. 12.1b).
- Exsanguinate the arm using a sterile Esmarch bandage (Fig. 12.2).
- Make the skin incision and use bipolar diathermy to cauterize visible vessels.

- Use blunt dissection with scissors to divide the subcutaneous fat down to the deep fascia. Identify and protect any braches of the medical antebrachial cutaneous nerves that cross the incision (Fig. 12.3a).

Procedure

- Identify the ulnar nerve lying posterior to the medial epicondyle. This is usually palpable and it can be "rolled" beneath your fingers.
- Release the ulnar nerve in the cubital tunnel. Begin by opening the cubital tunnel so that you can visibly see the nerve. It is sometimes easier to find the ulnar nerve distally between the two heads of flexor carpi ulnaris muscle (FCU) (Fig. 12.3b).
- Once the ulnar nerve has been identified, it should be released proximally and distally using sharp dissection. Distally, the nerve is released as it passes between the two heads of the FCU muscle (Fig. 12.4a). Take care when dividing the muscle to preserve the muscular nerve branches. There is often a sharp crescent of fascia (arcuate ligament) distally which should be divided (Fig. 12.4b).
- Release the ulnar nerve proximally. In some individuals, an anomalous muscle (anconeus epitrochlearis) lies over the ulnar nerve as it passes from the medial epicondyle to the triceps and olecranon – this should be divided. Ensure the ulnar nerve is released proximally to the medial intermuscular septum (Fig. 12.5).
- Ensure the nerve is not compressed by any fascial constrictions. Divide if present (Figs. 12.6a, b).

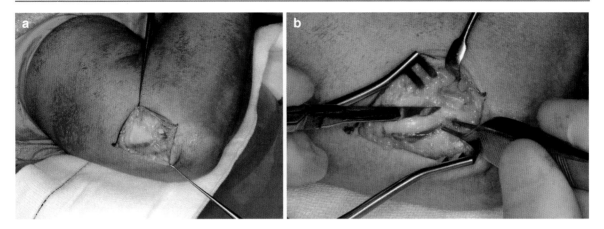

Fig. 12.3 (**a**) Skin incision with dissection of subcutaneous fat. Identify and protect any large sensory branches of the medial antebrachial cutaneous nerves if present. These are usually found distal to the medial epicondyle. (**b**) The ulnar nerve is released using sharp dissection. The medial triceps muscle is visible posteriorly adjacent to the forceps and the fascia over the FCU muscle is seen distally

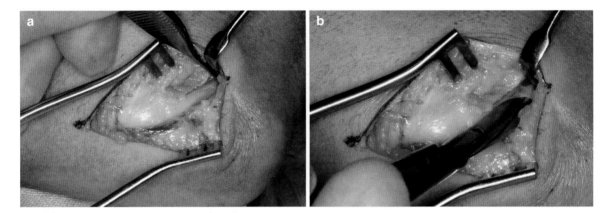

Fig. 12.4 (**a**) The ulnar nerve is released distally between the two heads of the FCU muscle.(**b**) A fascial band (the arcuate ligament) is clearly seen between the two heads of the FCU muscle. This should be divided

- Once the nerve has been released, check its stability by fully flexing the elbow and observing the ulnar nerve. If the nerve remains in the ulnar groove behind the medial epicondyle, you may choose to end the procedure (an in situ ulnar nerve release). If the ulnar nerve subluxes anteriorly riding over the medial epicondyle, you should proceed to an anterior transposition (Fig. 12.7).
- The ulnar nerve has to be fully mobilized before it is transposed. Use sharp dissection and only handle the nerve by the epineurium using fine-toothed forceps. Preserve the intraneural blood vessel plexus as much as possible. The nerve should be mobilized from proximal to the intermuscular septum to within the muscle of FCU.

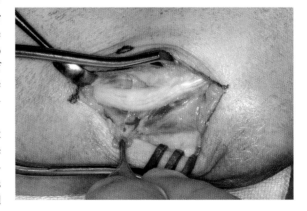

Fig. 12.5 The nerve is released proximally to beyond the medial intermuscular septum

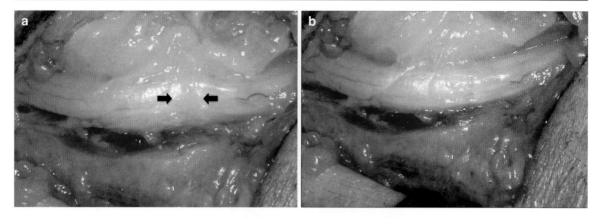

Fig. 12.6 (**a**) There is a fascial band compressing the ulnar nerve behind the medial epicondyle (*arrows*). (**b**) The fascial band in Fig. 1.9 has been divided

Fig. 12.7 The stability of the ulnar nerve is assessed. The ulnar nerve is shown in extension (*left*) and flexion (*right*). In flexion, the ulnar nerve subluxes anteriorly over the medial epicondyle indicating that it is unstable and an anterior transposition is required

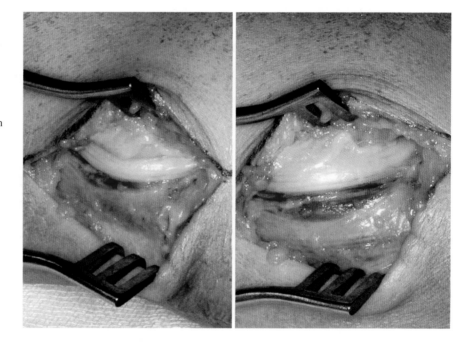

- Elevate the anterior soft tissues off the medial epicondyle and anteriorly at the level of the deep fascia to allow the nerve to lie on the medial epicondyle. Sharp dissection is important to reduce scarring. Transpose the ulnar nerve (Fig. 12.8).
- The inferior part of the medial intermuscular septum will be seen pressing on the ulnar nerve now that it has been transposed, and this is excised (Fig. 12.9a, b).
- Ensure that the ulnar nerve lies freely in its new position, and there are no kinks with elbow flexion

and extension. If it does not, this is usually because it has been completely mobilized proximally and distally.
- Attach the fascial layer of the anterior elevated soft tissues onto the fascia of the medial epicondyle with 4/0 Vicryl (Fig. 12.10a, b). This creates an anterior pocket to contain the ulnar nerve. Check that the nerve remains freely with full elbow flexion and extension, and you have not created any new compression.

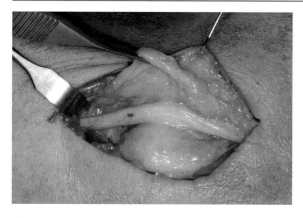

Fig. 12.8 The ulnar nerve has been mobilized with sharp dissection and the soft tissue elevated off the medial epicondyle to create a space for the ulnar nerve to be transposed

Closure

- Skin is closed in this case using a single subcuticular 3/0 Prolene suture (Fig. 12.11).
- Dress with petroleum jelly gauze, dressing gauze, velband, and a crepe bandage (Fig. 12.12).
- Release the tourniquet and elevate in a Bradford sling.

Postoperative Rehabilitation

- Encourage immediate finger mobilisation and elevate in a sling for 48 h
- Simple analgesia with paracetamol if required

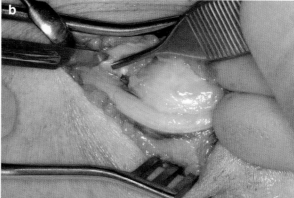

Fig. 12.9 (**a**) The medial intermuscular septum can be seen proximal to the medial epicondyle (*arrows*). This forms a sharp edge which kinks the ulnar nerve when it is transposed. (**b**) Part of the distal medial intermuscular septum is excised to permit the transposed ulnar nerve to lie freely

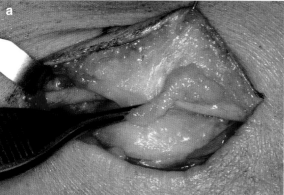
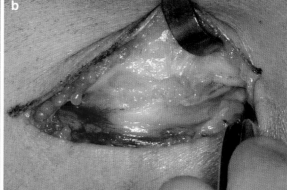

Fig. 12.10 (**a** and **b**) The anterior tissues that were elevated are attached to the medial epicondyle to leave the ulnar nerve in a "pocket" anteriorly

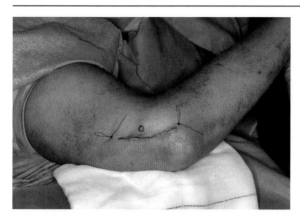

Fig. 12.11 Wound closure with a single subcuticular 3/0 Prolene suture

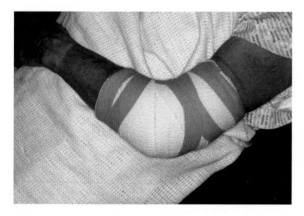

Fig. 12.12 Postoperative dressing and bandage shown after tourniquet removal

Outpatients Follow-up

- 2 weeks:
  - Suture and dressing removal
- 6 weeks:
  - Ensure symptoms are improving
  - Advice on scar massage with moisturiser (Fig. 20)
- Routine follow-up after this is not usually required.

Further Reading

Mackinnon SE. Comparative clinical outcomes of submuscular and subcutaneous transposition of the ulnar nerve for cubital tunnel syndrome. J Hand Surg Am. 2009;34(8):1574–5.

Macadam SA, Gandhi R, Bezuhly M, et al. Simple decompression versus anterior subcutaneous and submuscular transposition of the ulnar nerve for cubital tunnel syndrome: a meta-analysis. J Hand Surg Am. 2008;33(8):1314.

Gellman H. Compression of the ulnar nerve at the elbow: cubital tunnel syndrome. Instr Course Lect. 2008;57:187–97.

Elhassan B, Steinmann SP. Entrapment neuropathy of the ulnar nerve. J Am Acad Orthop Surg. 2007;15(11):672–81.

Lateral Collateral Ligament Reconstruction for Posterolateral Rotatory Instability of the Elbow

13

Panagiotis Stavlas and Christos Sinopidis

Indications

- Symptomatic chronic posterolateral rotatory instability (PLRI) of the elbow.
- The operative management focuses on the reconstruction of the lateral ulnar collateral band of the lateral ligament complex of the elbow which passes from the lateral epicondyle to the supinator crest of the ulna, using palmaris longus autograft.

Preoperative Planning

Clinical Assessment

- The diagnosis remains mainly a clinical one.
- Previous history of elbow trauma or surgery of the lateral elbow.
- Test varus and valgus instability of the elbow in 30° and 90° of flexion.
- Test valgus instability with the forearm pronated (testing in supination may give a false positive result in the presence of PLRI).
- Positive table-top relocation test.
- Positive chair sign.

P. Stavlas (✉)
Department of Trauma and Orthopaedics,
'Thriassio' General Hospital,
Elefsina, Greece
e-mail: stavlaspanagiotis@yahoo.gr

C. Sinopidis
'St. Luke's' Hospital,
Thessaloniki, Greece

- Positive lateral pivot-shift test under general anesthesia (Fig. 13.1a, b).

Radiological Assessment

- High-quality anteroposterior (AP) and lateral radiographs of the elbow.
- Usually, there are no radiographic pathological findings.

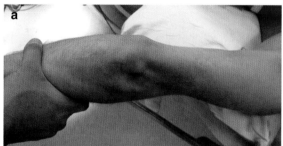

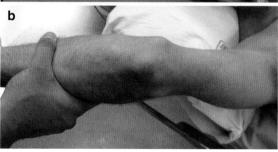

Fig. 13.1 (**a** and **b**) Lateral pivot-shift test for PLRI of the elbow joint. (**a**) The ulnohumeral joint is subluxed. Note the prominent radial head and the sulcus at the radiocapitellar joint. (**b**) The radial head has been reduced in the radiocapitellar joint during further flexion of the elbow

P.V. Giannoudis (ed.), *Practical Procedures in Elective Orthopaedic Surgery*,
DOI 10.1007/978-0-85729-820-1_13, © Springer-Verlag London Limited 2012

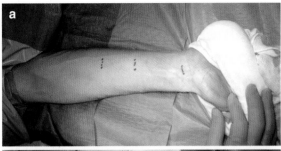
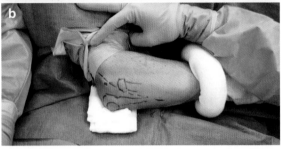

Fig. 13.2 (**a**) Skin incisions marking for the palmaris longus tendon harvest. (**b**) Lateral elbow planned skin incision (*dotted line*)

- However, examine for any posterior radial head location in relation to the capitellum on the lateral projection.
- Look for any avulsion fracture of the origin or insertion of the lateral ligament complex of the elbow.
- Look for any coronoid process fracture.
- MRI arthrography of the elbow is helpful when performed by an experienced musculoskeletal radiologist.

Operative Treatment

Anesthesia

- General anesthesia (interscalene block may additionally be used for the early postoperative period)
- Prophylactic antibiotics as per local hospital protocol
- Application of a pneumatic tourniquet to the upper arm

Table and Equipment

- Radiolucent arm table
- Suture anchors

Patient Positioning

- The patient is positioned supine, with the arm abducted and internally rotated on the arm table.

Draping and Surgical Approach

- Prepare the skin over arm, elbow, forearm, and hand with usual antiseptic solutions.
- Draw the skin incision planes using a skin marker (Fig. 13.2a, b).

Harvest and Preparation of Palmaris Longus Autograft

- Make a small (1–2 cm) transverse skin incision over the proximal flexion wrist crease. Locate and isolate the palmaris longus tendon at the ulnar side of the flexor carpi radialis tendon (Fig. 13.3a).
- Pulling on the tendon reveals its course on the distal and middle third of the forearm.
- Make a second small transverse skin incision over the tendon, 10 cm proximal to the first one (Fig. 13.3b). Locate and isolate again the palmaris longus tendon through this incision. Cut its distal end in the first incision and pull it subcutaneously through the second one.
- Make a third small transverse skin incision at the anticipated musculotendinous junction of the tendon, approximately 10 cm proximal to the second incision. Pull the tendon subcutaneously through this incision (Fig. 13.3c) and cut it just proximal to its musculotendinous junction.
- Remove any remaining muscle fibers from the proximal part of the tendon graft.
- The graft is folded along its long axis (making two equal length strands).
- Suture these two strands together using nonabsorbable (Ethibond No. 2) running sutures and apply 4–5 cycles of manual preconditioning of the graft (Fig. 13.4).
- Place the graft in a normal saline impregnated swab at the instrumentation table.
- Irrigate the wounds and close the skin.
- If palmaris longus tendon is not available, plantaris tendon, semitendinosus tendon, or triceps fascia can be used instead.

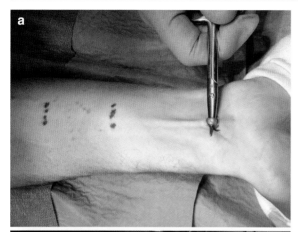

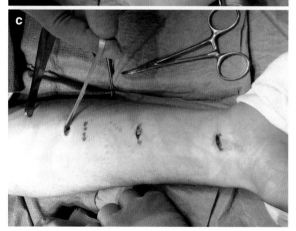

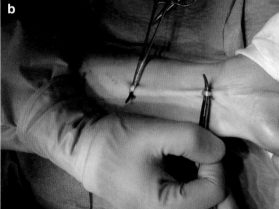

Fig. 13.3 Palmaris longus tendon harvest through (a) distal, (b) middle, and (c) proximal incision

Lateral Ulnar Collateral Ligament Reconstruction

- With the elbow flexed at 90° and the forearm in pronation, make a straight or slightly posteriorly curved incision at the lateral side of the

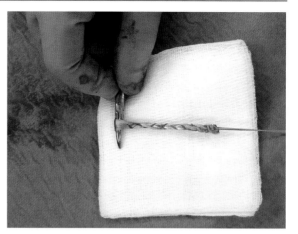

Fig. 13.4 The graft is folded along its long axis and braided with nonabsorbable sutures

elbow, starting 3 cm proximal to the lateral epicondyle and finishing at the lateral border of the ulna, 10 cm distal to the tip of the olecranon (Fig. 13.5a).
- Develop Kocher's interval, between anconeus and extensor carpi ulnaris, getting access to the radial compartment of the elbow (Fig. 13.5b).
- Release lateral collateral ligament complex (or scar tissue) from its insertion at the lateral epicondyle. Usually, the ligament complex may be torn or slack after the initial injury, and a discrete ligament band is not always apparent.
- Place a suture anchor at the center of the lateral epicondyle, where the ligament complex origins and the center of rotation of the joint is located (Fig. 13.6).
- Prepare the proximal part of the supinator crest of the ulna for fixation of the graft, using a small rasp for decortication. Test the isometry and tension of the planned graft placement, using a suture strand arising from the lateral epicondyle, locating its isometric insertion point at the supinator crest of the ulna (Fig. 13.7). Place a second suture anchor there.
- Suture one end of the graft at the lateral epicondyle anchor and the appropriate area of the other end of the graft at the supinator crest anchor, as tight as possible, with the elbow at 30° of flexion and the forearm in pronation (Fig. 13.8). Make sure that the graft passes over the radial head and is sutured in the supinator crest of the ulna under tension.

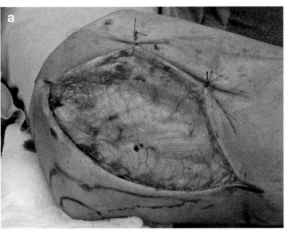
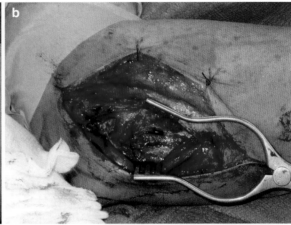

Fig. 13.5 (**a**) Skin incision. (**b**) Kocher's interval

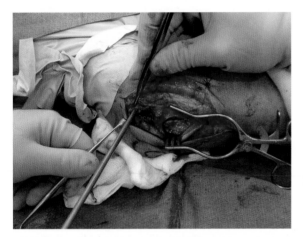

Fig. 13.6 Anchor placement at the lateral epicondyle

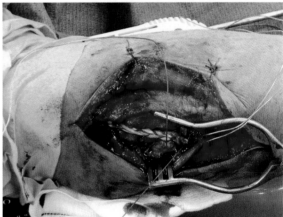

Fig. 13.8 Anchoring of the distal end of the graft using the sutures of the anchor that was placed at the supinator crest of the ulna

- Test the stability of the reconstructed lateral elbow joint and the tension of the graft applying several flexion–extension cycles in the elbow joint, keeping the forearm pronated (Fig. 13.9).
- Irrigate the wound thoroughly.
- Close the fascia and the rest of the wound in the usual way (Fig. 13.10).

Postoperative Treatment

- Apply a back slab with the elbow in 90° of flexion and the forearm pronated, for 24 h.
- Check neurovascular status of the limb.

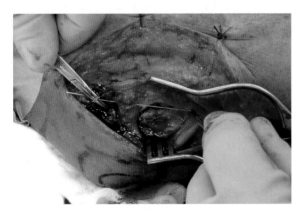

Fig. 13.7 Test of the isometry and tension of the planned graft placement, using a suture strand arising from the lateral epicondyle, locating its isometric insertion point at the supinator crest of the ulna

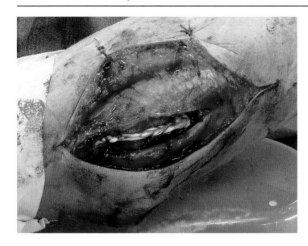

Fig. 13.9 Fixation and stability test

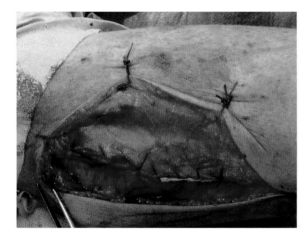

Fig. 13.10 Fascia closure

- Next day, a functional elbow brace is worn with the forearm in pronation for a total period of 6 weeks, permitting 60°-full flexion range of motion for the first 2 weeks, 30°-full flexion for the following 2 weeks, and full flexion–extension for the rest of the period.
- After that period, the brace is discontinued, and the patient is instructed for the next 6 weeks to start using his/her elbow in daily activities, avoiding excess strain at the reconstructed side, as during lifting weights with the shoulder abducted and the lateral part of elbow facing upwards.

Outpatients Follow-up

- Review patient at 2 weeks, 6 weeks, 12 weeks, 6 months, and 12 months, with radiographs on arrival of first visit.
- Consider return to full activities after 3 months.
- Consider return to contact sports at 6 months.

Further Reading

Charalambous CP, Stanley JK. Posterolateral rotatory instability of the elbow. J Bone Joint Surg Br. 2008;90:272–9.

Eygendaal D. Ligamentous reconstruction around the elbow using triceps tendon. Acta Orthop Scand. 2004;75: 516–23.

O'Driscoll SW. Classification and evaluation of recurrent instability of the elbow. Clin Orthop Relat Res. 2000; 370:34–43.

Olsen BS, Søjbjerg JO. The treatment of recurrent posterolateral instability of the elbow. J Bone Joint Surg Br. 2003; 85:342–6.

Sanchez-Sotelo J, Morrey BF, O'Driscoll SW. Ligamentous repair and reconstruction for posterolateral rotatory instability of the elbow. J Bone Joint Surg Br. 2005;87:54–61.

Elbow Arthroscopy

14

David Limb and Panagiotis Stavlas

Indications

- Diagnostic
  - The assessment of elbow pain or locking
- Therapeutic
  - Removal of loose bodies
  - Release of anterior capsular contractures (Fig. 14.1)
  - Debridement of early arthritic changes
- As expertise increases, the technique becomes applicable to a wider range of pathology, including radial head excision (Fig. 14.2a, b), epicondylitis, arthrofibrosis, reduction and fixation of fractures, and even ulnar nerve release.

Preoperative Planning

Clinical Assessment

- The clinical history usually defines the indication for surgery.
- Document the range of movement and the neurovascular status of the limb distal to the elbow. Arthroscopic entry into the stiff joint is predictably more difficult.

D. Limb (✉)
Leeds General Infirmary,
Leeds, UK
e-mail: d.limb@leevds.ac.uk

P. Stavlas
Orthopaedic Surgeon, Department of Trauma and Orthopaedics,
'Thriassio' General Hospital, Elefsina, Greece

Radiological Assessment

- Plain X-rays may show early osteophyte formation amenable to arthroscopic excision. It is important to know about any distortion of anatomy caused by trauma.
- CT or MR arthrography may be used to investigate locking (not plain CT or MRI – it is impossible to tell if cartilage or bone fragments are "loose" on imaging without contrast except in the case of MRI in the presence of an elbow effusion).

Operative Technique

- The procedure can be carried out supine, lateral, or prone.
- Equipment requirements are for the arthroscopy system and camera, the fluid flow system, and instruments to work within the joint (Fig. 14.3a, b).

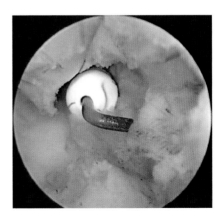

Fig. 14.1 Arthroscopic image of anterior capsular release

P.V. Giannoudis (ed.), *Practical Procedures in Elective Orthopaedic Surgery*,
DOI 10.1007/978-0-85729-820-1_14, © Springer-Verlag London Limited 2012

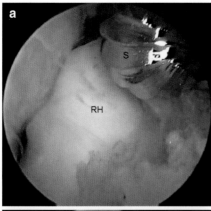

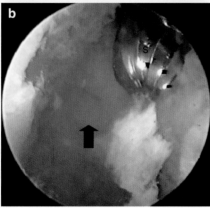

Fig. 14.2 (**a**) Radial head (*RH*) excision with a shaver (*S*), (**b**) After excision (*arrow* indicates the space created)

- A standard 6-mm arthroscope can be used – smaller scopes are easier to insert and maneuver but give a smaller field of view.
- A 6-mm scope used for shoulder arthroscopy is often used with a high-flow sheath to facilitate fluid management with an arthroscopic pump. The external diameter of these sheaths is 8 or 9 mm – too bulky for many elbows. A high-flow sheath is therefore not used.
- High fluid flows are not required, particularly if a tourniquet is used. Gravity inflow with or without a hand pump chamber for temporary increases in flow or pressure are usually adequate.

Anesthesia

- The procedure can be carried out under regional and/or general anesthesia.

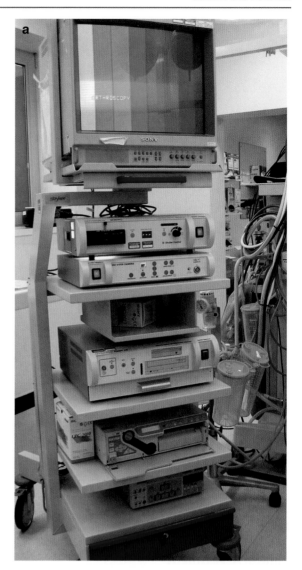

Fig. 14.3 (**a**) Arthroscopy system and camera. (**b**) Fluid flow system

Positioning and Equipment

- For the lateral position, the upper arm is allowed to rest on an arm holder projecting from the table. Patient position should allow equipment inserted through posterior portals (Fig. 14.4a).
- A tourniquet is applied and the time noted.

Draping and Surgical Approach

- Prepare the skin of the hand, forearm, and upper arm to the level of the tourniquet using your usual antiseptic

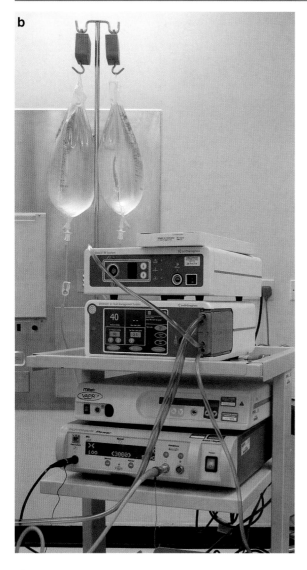

Fig. 14.3 (continued)

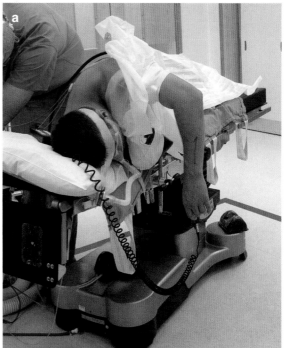

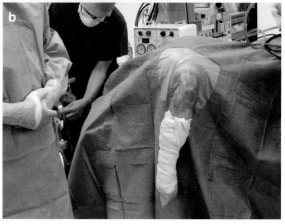

Fig. 14.4 (**a**) Lateral patient position with the arm rested on an arm holder. (**b**) Preparation of the skin and draping

solutions (e.g., aqueous povidone-iodine). Use an upper-extremity exclusion drape (Fig. 14.4b).

- The "soft spot" is palpated anterior to a line connecting the lateral epicondyle with the olecranon, which marks the radiocapitellar joint (Fig. 14.5).
- Using a large-bore needle, approximately 25–30 mL of saline is injected through the soft spot into the joint until slight resistance is felt. If the elbow is at 90° as injection takes place, the arm is observed to begin extending as the capsule distends (Fig. 14.6).
- A short incision is made at the lateral entry point through skin only (Fig. 14.7). There are various

identified portals posterior to the course of the radial nerve – a stab incision 2 cm distal and 1 cm anterior to the lateral epicondyle or 1 cm distal and 2 cm anterior to the same landmark allows safe access to the joint (Fig. 14.8a–c).

- Dissection beneath the level of the skin is done gently by spreading a clip (Fig. 14.9a). Once the joint capsule is reached, the arthroscope sheath with a conical (but not sharp) obturator can be inserted, aiming to an imaginary point halfway between the medial and lateral epicondyles (Fig. 14.9b).

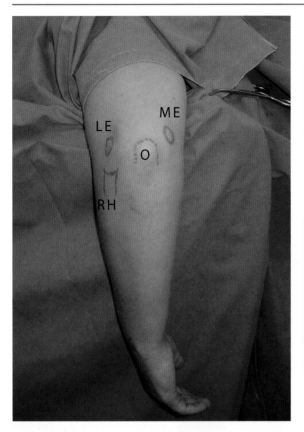

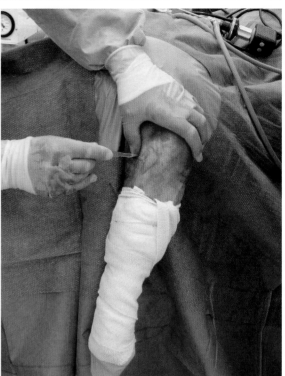

Fig. 14.7 A short incision is made at the lateral entry point through skin only

Fig. 14.5 The patient has been placed in the lateral decubitus position with the elbow flexed over a post, and the olecranon (*O*), radial head (*RH*), lateral (*LE*), and medial (*ME*) epicondyles have been delineated (*red marks*)

Portals

Anterior Compartment Portals

- *Lateral side*
  - *Proximal anterolateral portal.* This is the primary arthroscope (diagnostic) portal. It is located 2 cm proximal and 2 cm anterior to the lateral epicondyle (Fig. 14.8a). The brachialis muscle serves as a cushion to protect the vulnerable neurovascular structures.
  - *Standard anterolateral portal.* It is located 1 cm distal and 3 cm anterior to the lateral epicondyle, in close proximity to the posterior interosseous nerve.
  - *Midanterolateral portal.* It is located 2 cm directly anterior to the lateral epicondyle.
- *Medial side*
  - *Proximal anteromedial portal.* It is located 2 cm proximal and 2 cm anterior to the medial epicondyle (Fig. 14.8b). It is used as a working portal and usually is established using a switching rod (inside–out technique), which is inserted through the anterolateral portal (Fig. 14.10).

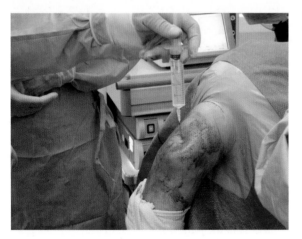

Fig. 14.6 Using a large-bore needle, approximately 25–30 mL of saline is injected from the soft spot into the joint

- A "flashback" of fluid from the distended joint confirms entry. The obturator is removed and the camera inserted.

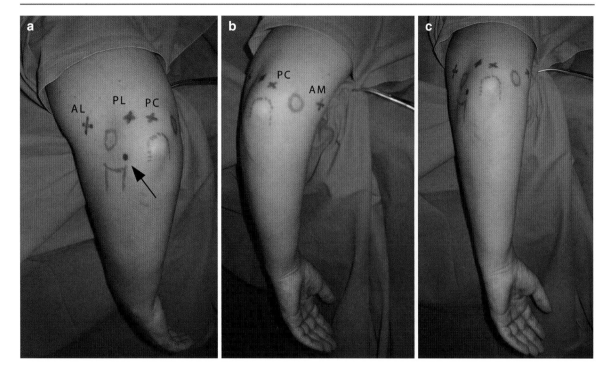

Fig. 14.8 (**a**) The "soft-spot" (*arrow*), the proximal anterolateral (*AL*), posterocentral (*PC*), and superior posterolateral (*PL*) portals (*blue marks*). (**b**) The proximal anteromedial (*AM*) and the posterocentral (*PC*) portals (*blue marks*), and (**c**) The relation between the anterior and posterior portals

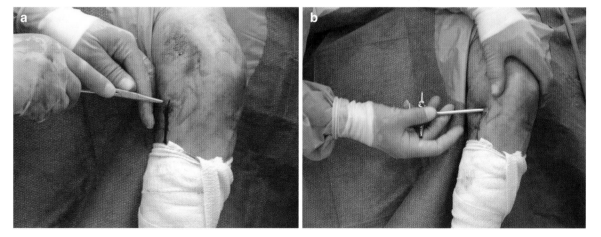

Fig. 14.9 (**a**) Dissection beneath the level of the skin is done gently by spreading a clip. (**b**) Insertion of the arthroscope sheath with a conical (but not sharp) obturator

– *Standard anteromedial portal.* It is located 2 cm distal and 2 cm anterior to the medial epicondyle. The ulnar nerve, brachial artery, and median nerve are at risk when establishing and using this portal.

Posterior Compartment Portals

• *"Soft-spot" portal.* It is located in the triangle formed between the radial head, the tip of the olecranon, and the lateral epicondyle (the palpable "soft-spot" area) of the posterolateral elbow joint (Fig. 14.8a). It is used before any other portal placement for needle access and joint distention.

• *Straight posterior or posterocentral portal.* It is located 3 cm proximal to the tip of the olecranon (Fig. 14.8a, b). It is used primarily for visualization of the medial and lateral posterior compartments and of the olecranon fossa.

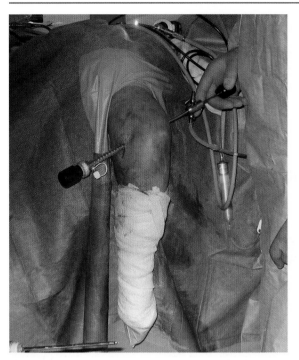

Fig. 14.10 Inside–out technique for the proximal anteromedial portal

- *Superior posterolateral portal.* It is located 1–2 cm proximal and 1–2 cm lateral to the previously established straight posterior portal. Alternatively it can be placed anywhere in the posterolateral gutter (outside the triceps tendon), at a level 2–3 cm proximal to the tip of the olecranon (Fig. 14.8a).

The Surgical Procedure

- Once in the joint, a systematic inspection of all compartments takes place (Fig. 14.11). A probe can be passed through an anteromedial portal, situated 2 cm distal and 2 cm anterior to the medial epicondyle. Alternatively this portal can be made from the inside out if a switching stick is passed up the scope and directed to the posterior capsule.
- Access to the posterior compartments is gained lateral to the triceps tendon or directly through it.
- Once loose bodies are identified, they can be removed. Small loose bodies can be extracted along the tract of the instrument. Larger ones may need a small incision once they are in a subcutaneous position.

Closure

- Wounds are closed with steristrips and a "wool and crepe" bandage that is removed after 48 h.

Postoperative Care and Rehabilitation

- After diagnostic arthroscopy or removal of loose bodies, the bulky dressing can be removed after 48 h and the steristrips by 2 weeks.

Complications

- Nerve injury. Overall, the rate of complications after elbow arthroscopy has fallen over the past two decades as experience has increased. However, there is a significant learning curve, and it is not an operation for the occasional operator. Nerve injury risk is minimized by avoiding prolonged tourniquet times, taking care with padding the surfaces the arm rests on, and paying heed to careful portal siting, avoiding sharp dissection beneath the skin entry point.
- Infection, fortunately rare as the elbow is washed out throughout the procedure.
- Poor views – do not be afraid to abandon the procedure rather than trying to work with inadequate views when an instrumented procedure is being carried out. Intra-articular retractors are available though often require additional portals themselves.
- Compartment syndrome is a risk, and for this reason, pressurization of the fluid should be avoided and a fluid outflow should be kept open.

Results

- Initially complication rates were high, with reported rates of temporary nerve palsy of up to 30%. Fortunately this is now much less with experience, though temporary neurological symptoms may occur in up to 5%, depending on the procedure.
- For removal of loose bodies, the arthroscopic technique is better than open surgery, in which even an

Fig. 14.11 (a–d) Synovectomy and loose body removal of the anterior compartment of the elbow. (*T* trochlea, *CP* coronoid process, *Cap* capitellum, *RH* radial head, *L* loose body). (e, f) Synovectomy of the olecranon fossa (*OF*) and visualization of the ulnohumeral joint

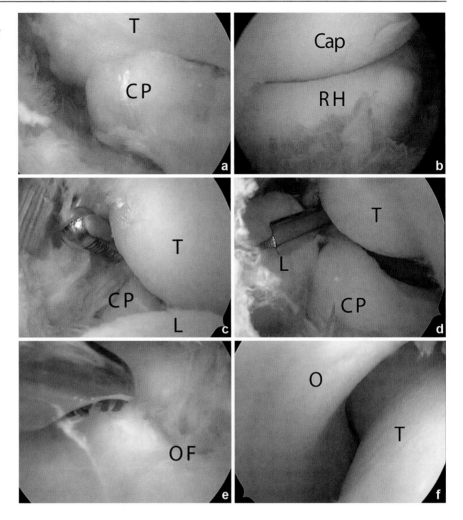

extensive exposure does not give access to all recesses of this complexly shaped joint.

Follow-up

- The patient is reviewed at 2 weeks, and the wound is checked, along with elbow range of movement, which is compared to pre-operative findings. At this point the pathology discovered and treated can be discussed with the patient.

Further Reading

Dodson CC, Nho SJ, Williams III RJ. Elbow arthroscopy. J Am Acad Orthop Surg. 2008;16(10):574–85.

Steinmann SP. Elbow arthroscopy: where are we now? Arthroscopy. 2007;23(11):1231–6.

Steinmann SP, King GJ, Savoie III FH. Arthroscopic treatment of the arthritic elbow. Instr Course Lect. 2006;55:109–17.

Noonburg GE, Baker Jr CL. Elbow arthroscopy. Instr Course Lect. 2006;55:87–93.

Total Elbow Arthroplasty

Panayotis N. Soucacos and Panagiotis Liantis

Introduction

- Total elbow arthroplasty (TEA) has proven to be a reliable joint replacement procedure that has a high degree of patient satisfaction.
- Aims:
  - Alleviate pain
  - Improve ROM
  - Restore stability
  - Eliminate joint stiffness
  - Correct flexion/contracture

Indications

- Severe pain, stiffness, and loss of function, non-corresponding at other treatment modalities, with radiological changes of joint destruction due to:
  - Rheumatoid arthritis
  - Osteoarthritis (Fig. 15.1a, b)
  - Post-traumatic arthritis
  - Hemophilic arthropathy
  - Severely damaged or torn soft tissues in the elbow resulting in instability

P.N. Soucacos (✉)
Academic Department of Trauma and Orthopaedic Surgery,
School of Medicine, University of Athens,
Athens, Greece
e-mail: psoukakos@ath.forthnet.gr

P. Liantis
Third Academic Department of Trauma and Orthopaedic Surgery,
School of Medicine, University of Athens,
Athens, Greece

- Malignancy in or around the elbow
- Poor results from previous elbow surgery
- Complex fracture of the elbow, even in the elderly (Fig. 15.2a, b)
- Distal humerus malunions and nonunions

Contraindications

- Neuropathic joint.
- Flaccid paralysis of the upper extremity.
- Non-restorable function of the biceps and triceps.
- Poor soft tissue coverage.
- Presence of infection at the elbow.
- Poor patient compliance with activity and weight-lifting restrictions.

Risks

- Intraoperatively:
  - Nerve damage, especially the ulnar nerve
  - Blood vessel damage
  - Fracture
- Postoperatively:
  - Dislocation of the prosthesis
  - Loosening of the implant over time
  - Allergic reaction to the implant
  - Fracture of the prosthesis is uncommon, but if it occurs, results of revision surgery are reasonably satisfactory
  - Stiffness or instability of the joint
  - Detachment of the triceps tendon
  - Pain

Fig. 15.1 (**a**) AP and
(**b**) lateral X-rays of an
elbow with osteoarthritis

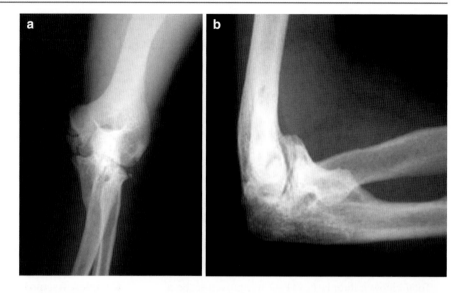

Fig. 15.2 (**a**) AP
and (**b**) lateral X-rays of a
complex fracture of the
elbow in an elderly patient
with osteoporosis

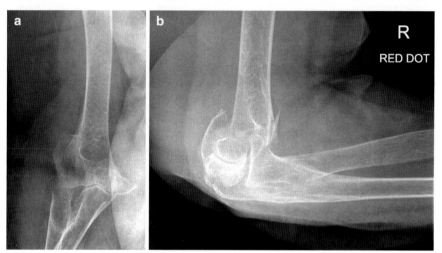

Radiological Assessment

- Radiographs:
  - A recent AP and lateral X-rays of the elbow
- CT and MRI:
  - CT and MRI may be needed in cases radiographs do not provide adequate detail of the elbow joint. CT and MRI provide also three-dimensional images of the area

Scoring System

- The most widely used outcome score is Mayo elbow performance score (MEPS) (Table 15.1).

Design Goals

- Re-establish anatomy.
- Restore joint mechanics.
- Increase articular surface contact.
- Evolve instrumentation.

Implant Selection

- Total elbow designs can be divided in several broad categories.

Table 15.1 Mayo elbow performance score (*MEPS*)

Pain (max: 45 points)	
None	45 points
Mild	30 points
Moderate	15 points
Severe	0 points
Range of motion (max: 20 points)	
Arc > 100°	20 points
Arc 50–100°	15 points
Arc < 50°	5 points
Stability (max: 10 points)	
Stable	10 points
Moderately unstable	5 points
Grossly unstable	0 points
Function (max: 25 points)	
Able to comb hair	5 points
Able to feed oneself	5 points
Able to perform personal hygiene tasks	5 points
Able to put on shirt	5 points
Able to put on shoes	5 points
Mean total (max: 100 points)	
Score >90	Excellent
Score 75–89	Good
Score 60–74	Fair
Score < 60	Poor

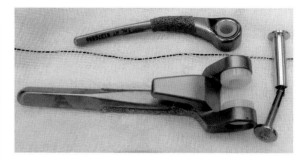

Fig. 15.3 Implants for a linked total elbow arthroplasty

Unlinked Total Elbow Arthroplasties

Minimally Constrained or Semi-Constrained

- Unlinked or unconstrained implants are not mechanically linked but rely on matching shapes of the bearing surfaces.
- Unlinked designs require competent soft tissue constraints and adequate bone stock length to yield a stable arthroplasty.
- Be preferred in younger patients who may need later revision surgery.
- Decreases loosening at the bone-cement interface but carries a greater risk for instability.

Convertible Implants

Combined Linked-Unlinked

- These prostheses have the capacity to be inserted in an unlinked or a linked fashion.
- Benefits from both designs.

Linked Versus Unlinked Total Elbow Arthroplasties

- Patients without increased bone destruction and ligamentous incompetency are candidates for unlinked arthroplasty.
- Patient with insufficient bone stock, advanced osseous deformity, gross instability, and capsuloligamentous insufficiency are candidates for linked arthroplasty.

Linked Total Elbow Arthroplasties

Semi-Constrained

- Linked implants are coupled together with pins or snap fit (Fig. 15.3).
- Degree of laxity in the medial, lateral, and rotational planes.
- Simulates the loose hinge of normal elbow kinematics.
- Indicated:
  - In later stages of rheumatoid arthritis, post-traumatic arthritis, and osteoarthritis where increased bone destruction and ligamentous incompetency exist
  - For complex displaced intra-articular fractures that are not adequately reduced by fracture internal fixation techniques, particularly in elderly patients with osteoporotic bone
  - For distal humerus malunions and nonunions
- Lower rate of instability.
- Higher rate of aseptic loosening.

Fig. 15.4 Trays with instruments according to the implant selected

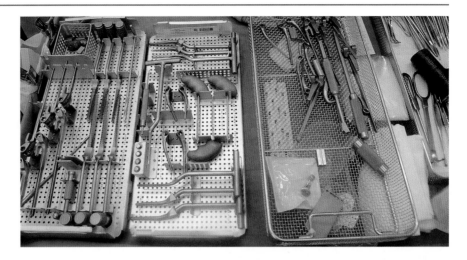

Operative Treatment

Anesthesia

- General anesthesia is administered for the procedure, but regional anesthesia with sedation can also be employed.
- The majority of patients first undergo placement of an indwelling auxiliary or infraclavicular catheter for postoperative pain control.

Table and Equipment

- A radiolucent table is advisable to be used, in case that intraoperative X-rays are going to be needed.
- Instrumentation, trial, and implants according to the implant selected (Fig. 15.4).

Patient Positioning

- Place the patient in a supine or lateral position:
  - For the supine position, lay the affected arm across the patient's chest to give access to the posterior aspect of the joint. A bolster or a sand bag may be placed under the scapula to elevate the operative site
  - For the lateral position, the upper arm is allowed to rest on an arm holder projecting from the table (Fig. 15.5)
- An upper arm tourniquet is applied, and the time is noted.

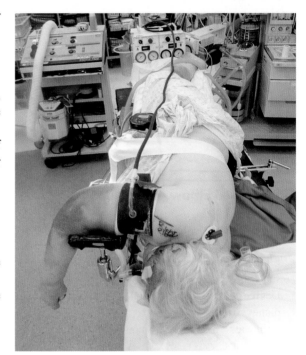

Fig. 15.5 Lateral position

Draping and Surgical Approach

- Prepare the skin of the hand, forearm, and upper arm to the level of the tourniquet using your usual antiseptic solutions (e.g., aqueous povidone iodine) (Fig. 15.6a).
- Use an upper extremity exclusion drape (Fig. 15.6b).
- A posterior skin incision is the preferred approach for total elbow arthroplasty. A posterolateral Kocher

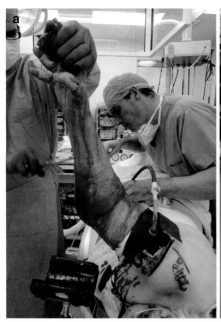
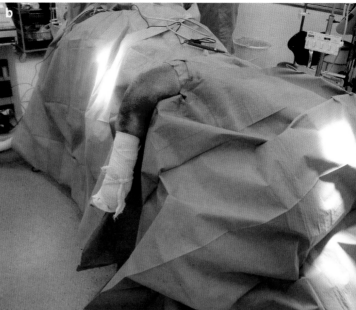

Fig. 15.6 (**a**) Skin preparation with antiseptic solution.(**b**) Upper limb draping

approach is the most often used for unlinked implant surgery.

- Mark a longitudinal posterior incision – curve it to the radial side of the olecranon.
- Dissect the subcutaneous tissues.
- The ulnar nerve must be identified at the cubital tunnel, mobilized and protected throughout the surgical procedure. Nerve transpositioning is often necessary (Fig. 15.7).
- Dissect triceps aponeurosis (Fig. 15.8a).
- Invert a V-shaped flap of the triceps aponeurosis (Fig. 15.8b). Leave the triceps tendon attached distally to the tip of the olecranon.
- Split the triceps muscle longitudinally, and expose the distal humerus subperiosteally.
- Rotate the forearm laterally to allow exposure of the distal humerus (Fig. 15.8c).

Implants Positioning

- Begin preparing the distal humerus.
- Using an oscillating saw, remove the midportion of the trochlea.
- Prepare the medullary canal with a twist reamer and place the alignment stem with a T-handle (Fig. 15.9a).
- Apply the cutting block and proceed with distal humerus osteotomy.

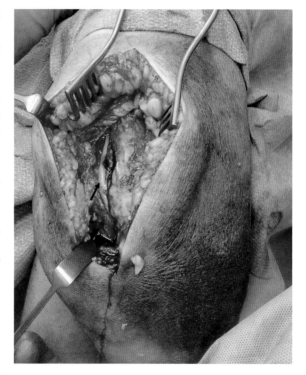

Fig. 15.7 Ulnar nerve (*arrow*)

- Rasp the subchondral bone (Fig. 15.9b).
- Finish with a "U"-shaped cut in the humerus.
- Continue with preparation of the ulna.

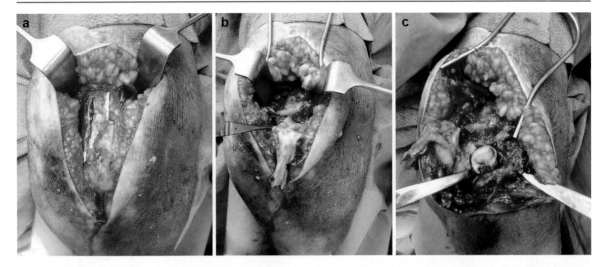

Fig. 15.8 (**a**) Triceps aponeurosis' dissection. (**b**) Inversion of a V-shaped flap of the triceps aponeusosis. (**c**) Forearm lateral rotation

Fig. 15.9 (**a**) Placement of alignment stem with a T-handle into humeral medullary canal. (**b**) Rasping the subchondral bone of distal humerus

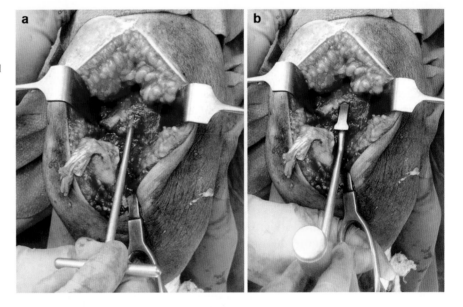

- Form a notch at the tip of the olecranon.
- Introduce reamers to the medullary canal (Fig. 15.10a) and rasps (Fig. 15.10b).
- A trial application should be performed (Figs. 15.11–15.13).
- Prior to cement application, prepare autograft from the bone removed with the osteotomies (Fig. 15.14a). Elevate humeral periosteum anterior to the distal humeral cortex and place the bone graft against the distal humerus beneath the soft tissue.
- Prepare the cement (Fig. 15.14b).

- Keep humeral and ulnar canal dry and apply cement with a cement gun with flexible tubing (Fig. 15.15a, b).
- Insert the final components (Fig. 15.16a). The two stems are joined with or without the hinge mechanism (Fig. 15.16b, c).

Closure

- Close the triceps aponeurosis (Fig. 15.17a–c).
- Drain is an option, and it has to be removed within 48 h.

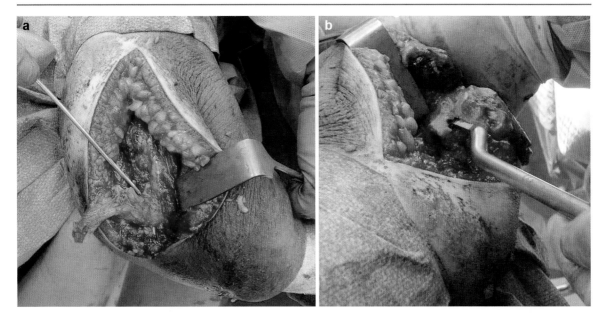

Fig. 15.10 (**a**) Intramedullary reamers into proximal ulna. (**b**) Rasping the subchondral bone of proximal ulna

Fig. 15.11 (**a**) Insertion of humeral trial implant (**b**) the component in place

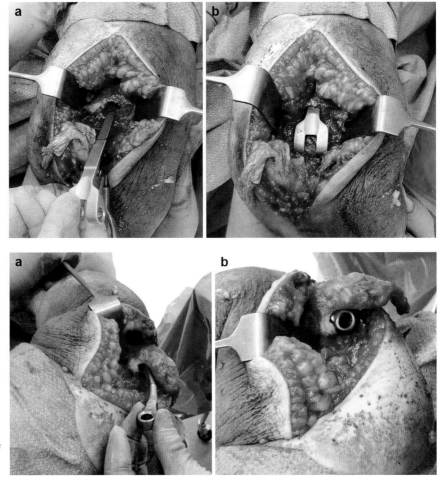

Fig. 15.12 (**a**) Insertion of the ulnar trial implant (**b**) the component in place

Fig. 15.13 (**a**) The two trial stems are joined with the hinge mechanism (**b**) the final appearance

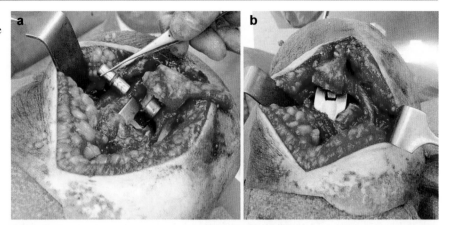

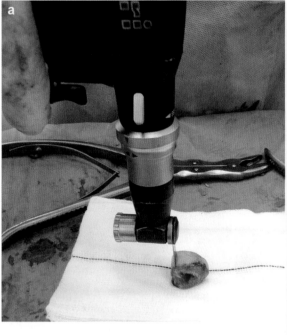

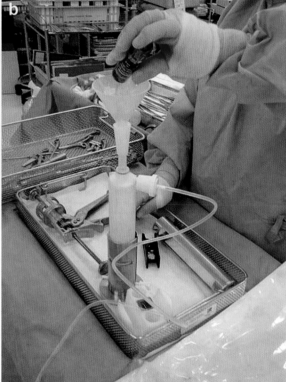

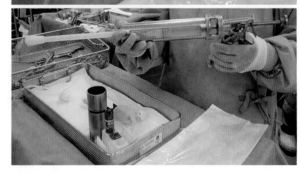

Fig. 15.14 (**a**) Graft preparation. (**b**) Cement preparation

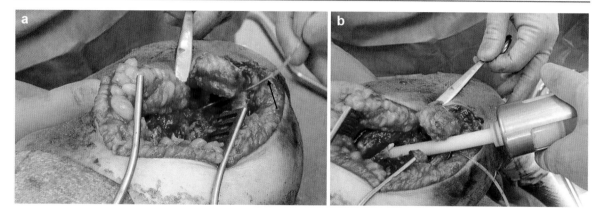

Fig. 15.15 (**a**) Keeping femoral and ulnar canal dry before cement application with a small tube (*arrow*). (**b**) Cement application with a cement gun

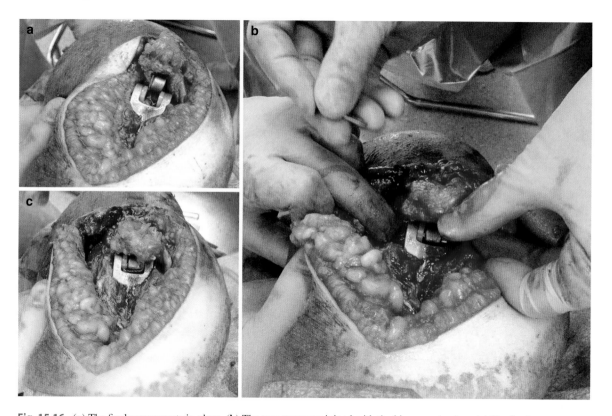

Fig. 15.16 (**a**) The final components in place. (**b**) The two stems are joined with the hinge mechanism. (**c**) The final outcome

- The wound is closed in layers (Fig. 15.18a, b).
- A bandage is applied to splint the arm for stability.
- Some surgeons apply a plaster cast with the elbow extended, others with the elbow at 90°. The plaster cast is usually removed at 48–72 h, and gentle mobilization is commenced.

Postoperative Management

- Postoperative AP and lateral X-rays (Fig. 15.19a, b) are necessary to control the good alignment of the prosthesis.
- The patient will stay in hospital for about 5–7 days.
- Elevate the elbow.

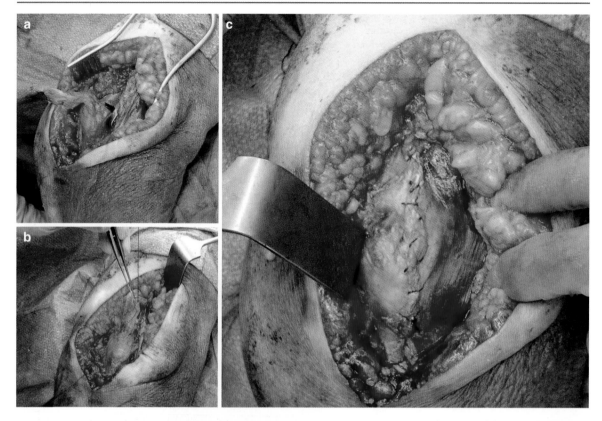

Fig. 15.17 (**a**) Appearance after insertion of components (**b**) triceps aponeurosis flap is pulled into place (**c**) triceps aponeurosis closure

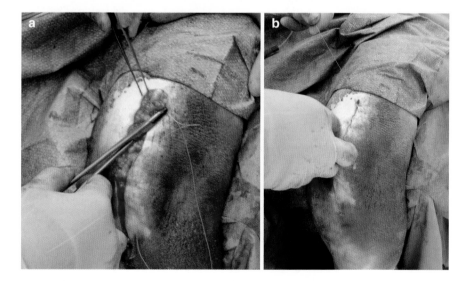

Fig. 15.18 (**a**) Wound's subcutaneous layer closure and (**b**) skin closure

- Routine antibiotic according to local protocols.
- Begin active and gentle passive range-of-motion exercises at 7–10 days.
- Protect triceps if detached for 6–8 weeks.

- Use night-time elbow extension splint for sleep in maximum extension to limit potential flexion contracture.
- Physiotherapy starts with gentle flexing exercises.

Fig. 15.19 Postoperative radiographs, (**a**) AP and (**b**) lateral

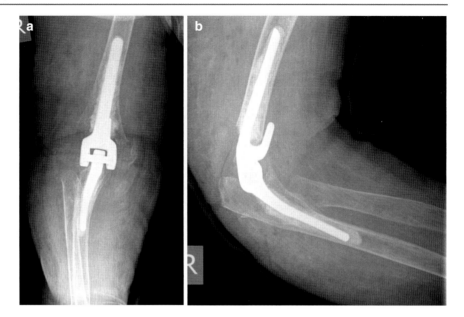

- The patient will need help with everyday activities, such as driving, shopping, bathing, meal preparation, and household chores, for up to 6 weeks.
- Some patients may begin to regain function of the elbow as soon as 12 weeks after surgery, although additional recovery can take up to a year.
- The patient should not lift more than about 2.5 kg with the operated arm, even when fully recovered.

Complication

- Complication rate 20–45%.
- Humeral, ulnar, radial head or component fracture.
- Periprosthetic fractures.
- Superficial or deep wound infection.
- Temporary or permanent nerve damage.
- Damage to blood vessels.
- Hematoma.
- Delayed would healing.
- Implant loosening, polyethylene wear, implant failure.
- Cardiovascular disorders including venous thrombosis, pulmonary embolism, or myocardial infarction.

Follow-up

- It is advisable to follow the patients up to a year postoperatively and every 5 years thereafter, unless GP's request.

Long-Term Patient Limitations

- Patients should avoid activities that involve impact (hammering, chopping wood, contact sports, sports with major risk of falls) or heavy loads (lifting of heavy weights, heavy resistance exercises). These activities may increase the chance of loosening, wear, or fracture.

Further Reading

King GJ. New frontiers in elbow reconstruction: total elbow arthroplasty. Instr Course Lect. 2002;51:43–51.

Little CP, Graham AJ, Carr AJ. Total elbow arthroplasty: a systematic review of the literature in the English language until the end of 2003. J Bone Joint Surg Br. 2005;87:437–44.

Morrey BF, An KN, Chao EYS. Functional evaluation of the elbow. In: Morrey BF, editor. The elbow and its disorders. 2nd ed. Philadelphia: W. B. Saunders; 1993. p. 86–9.

Peden JP, Morrey BF. Total elbow replacement for the management of the ankylosed or fused elbow. J Bone Joint Surg Br. 2008;90-B:1198–204.

Moro JK, King GJ. Total elbow arthroplasty in the treatment of posttraumatic conditions of the elbow. Clin Orthop Relat Res. 2000;370:102–14.

Wright TW, Wong AM, Jaffe R. Functional outcome comparison of semiconstrained and unconstrained total elbow arthroplasties. J Shoulder Elbow Surg. 2000;9:524–31.

Angst F, John M, Pap G, et al. Comprehensive assessment of clinical outcome and quality of life after total elbow arthroplasty. Arthritis Rheum. 2005;53:73–82.

Part III

Upper Extremity: Forearm – Wrist

Forearm Nonunions

16

Peter V. Giannoudis, Efthimios J. Karadimas, and Fragkiskos N. Xypnitos

Indications

- A nonunion should be revised if it:
  - Is painful.
  - Is related with underline infection.
  - Affects either the radius or the ulna or both forearm bones.
  - Is related with hardware (ORIF) failure.

Clinical Symptoms

- Pain localized over the nonunion site.
- Sometimes abnormal motion over the nonunion site can be indentified.

Preoperative Planning

Clinical Assessment

- Meticulous patient and injury history.
- Complete physical examination of the patient.

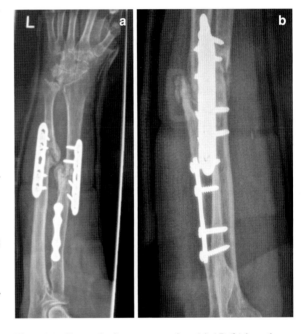

Fig. 16.1 X-ray of a forearm nonunion. (**a**) AP, (**b**) lateral

- Thorough examination of the extremity:
  - Evaluate the most painful site.
  - Neurovascular examination of the forearm and wrist.
  - Check for any residual sinus.

Radiological Assessment

- Plain AP/lateral X-rays is the first step of the investigation (Fig. 16.1a, b).
- In elusive cases, perform a high-resolution CT, which will provide useful information of the nonunion site (type of nonunion).

P.V. Giannoudis (✉)
Academic Department of Trauma and Orthopaedic Surgery, School of Medicine, University of Leeds, Leeds, UK
e-mail: pgiannoudi@aol.com

E.J. Karadimas
Department of Trauma and Orthopaedic Surgery, Leeds Teaching Hospitals NHS Trust, Leeds, UK

F.N. Xypnitos
Department of Trauma and Orthopaedics, Leeds Teaching Hospitals NHS Trust, Leeds, UK

P.V. Giannoudis (ed.), *Practical Procedures in Elective Orthopaedic Surgery*,
DOI 10.1007/978-0-85729-820-1_16, © Springer-Verlag London Limited 2012

Fig. 16.2 Small fragment set

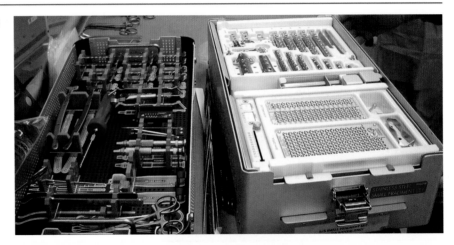

- MRI is also an option to investigate possible low-grade infection and assess the vascularity of the bony edges in cases where metal work is not present in situ.

Laboratory Tests

- Routine labs (FBC and biochemistry).
- If infection is suspected, evaluate the ESR, CRP.

Operative Treatment

Anaesthesia

- The procedure can be carried out under regional and/or general anaesthesia.
- Administration of prophylactic antibiotics is held until the acquisition of intraoperative cultures.

Table/Equipment

- Radiolucent table
- Imaging intensifier
- DVR and Small fragment sets (Fig. 16.2)
- Above elbow tourniquet
- Availability of bone grafts (consider autologous iliac crest graft, BMP-7, or RIA autograft)

Patient Positioning

- Supine position.
- The arm is positioned over a radiolucent side table for radius exposure (Fig. 16.3). For ulna exposure, the

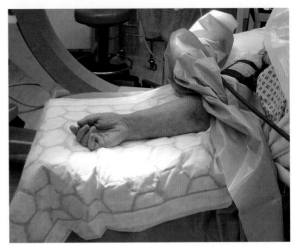

Fig. 16.3 The arm is positioned over a radiolucent side table

patient can be positioned either on the non-affected side or supine, with the hand flexed over his/her chest.

Marking and Draping

- Extensive skin preparation with the use of antiseptic solutions (alcoholic povidone/iodine) up to the level of the tourniquet. Extra care in the web spaces between the fingers.
- Sterile drape or a glove can be used to cover the fingers as an extra precaution.
- With the image intensifier, indentify the nonunion site and mark the incision.
- In cases of a revision surgery, it is advisable to use the incision of the first operation.
- Inflate humeral tourniquet to 250 mmHg.

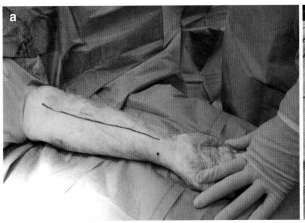
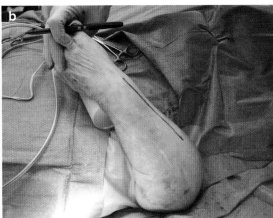

Fig. 16.4 (**a**) Skin marking for radius approach. (**b**) Skin marking for ulna approach

Surgical Exposure

- For radius
  - The skin incision line lies over the volar aspect of the forearm.
    Landmarks: groove between brachioradialis and distal biceps tendon proximally and styloid process of radius distally (Fig. 16.4a).
  - Make a straight skin incision.
  - Identify the flexor carpi radialis (FCR) tendon at the ulnar side and the brachioradialis at the radial side of the incision.
  - Incise the subcutaneous fascia between the FCR and the brachioradialis.
  - Care must be taken to protect the anterior cutaneous nerve of the forearm and the superficial radial nerve that run along the brachioradialis muscle as well as the radial artery.
  - Reflect FCR to the ulnar side and the brachioradialis to the radial side.
  - Following that, the pronator quadratus (PQ), the flexor digitorum sublimes (FDS), and the flexor pollicis longus (FPL) are exposed.
  - Subperiosteal elevation of the FPL and PQ. Strip them towards the ulna.
  - Proximally, release FDS, FDP, and pronator muscles from the volar radial aspect.
- For ulna
  - The skin incision line lies over the line connecting ulnar styloid process, and the tip of olecranon, directly over the subcutaneous border (Fig. 16.4b).

  - The deep incision is between extensor carpi ulnaris (posterior interosseous nerve) and the flexor carpi ulnaris (ulnar nerve).
- Usually the authors prefer to start with the radius exposure and fixation followed by the ulna.
- The bony edges of the nonunion site must be carefully trimmed, avoiding undesirable bone shortening. Small drill holes are advisable to be performed using the 2.5mm drill in order to open the medullary canal. Part of the available bone graft can be placed in the bony gap and packed, followed by implant positioning.

Implant Positioning

- The plate must be long enough to neutralize the torsional forces (at least six cortices in each main fragment).
- Pre-bend the plate to avoid developing a gap in the contralateral side.
- Place the appropriate dynamic compression plate and hold it in place with clamps (Fig. 16.5a).
- Place the first cortical screw in a neutral position, implementing the offset drill guide, without inserting it completely into the plate.
- The second screw should be placed eccentrically on the opposite site in a similar fashion.
- By tightening these two screws, compression is applied at the nonunion site.
- Continue by inserting the remaining screws (Fig. 16.5b).
- As soon as the fixation of the ulna is completed, the fixation of the radius must be inspected for any screw loosening.

Fig. 16.5 (**a**) The reduction forceps hold the plate in the appropriate position. (**b**) Measurement of screw length with the depth measurer

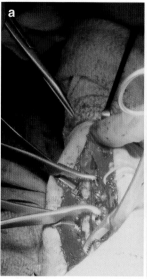
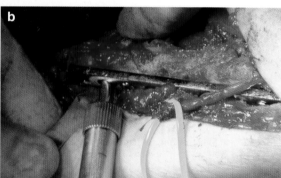

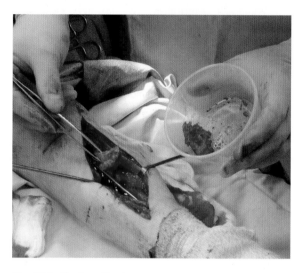

Fig. 16.6 Graft application

- In cases that the surgeon uses BMPs or other growth factors, drain is not advisable.
- Use 2/0 Vicryl interrupted sutures for closure of the subcutaneous layer.
- Use 3/0 Ethilon interrupted sutures or skin staples for skin closure.
- Wound dressing and wool application prior forearm's stabilization with an above elbow back slab.
- Be cautious not to apply the back slab tightly.

Postoperative Care/Rehabilitation

- Check neurological status.
- Elevation of the arm.
- Wound inspection within 48 h.
- Apply above elbow jig saw cast.
- Obtain radiographs AP/lateral (Fig. 16.7a, b).
- Retain the cast for 4 weeks followed by another two with a below elbow jig saw cast.
- After 6 weeks, the jig saw cast is removed and physiotherapy is commenced.

Complications

- Wound infection
- Compartment syndrome especially after prolonged tourniquet application
- Nonunion/high incidence in smokers.
- Radio–ulna synostosis

- Clinically assess alignment and rotation. Fluoroscopy documentation of implants position is advised prior to closure.
- The rest of bone graft and growth factors must be applied in the void and pressed (Fig. 16.6).

Closure

- Release tourniquet and check for any sources of bleeding.
- Irrigate wound with caution preserving the graft in place.

Fig. 16.7 Postoperative X-rays (**a**) AP and (**b**) lateral

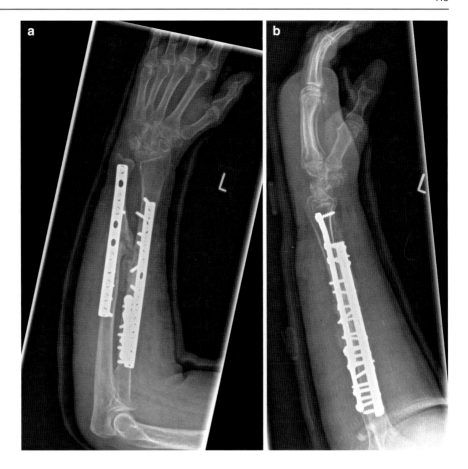

Follow-up

- Outpatients' follow-up at 4, 8, 12 weeks for clinical and radiological assessment (AP/lateral X-rays) and thereafter as indicated (i.e., 6 months).
- Discharged after bone consolidation is obtained clinically and radiologically.

Implant Removal

- It is not routinely performed.

Further Reading

Prasarn ML, Ouellette EA, Miller DR. Infected nonunions of diaphyseal fractures of the forearm. Arch Orthop Trauma Surg. 2010;130(7):867–73.

dos Reis FB, Faloppa F, Fernandes HJ, et al. Outcome of diaphyseal forearm fracture-nonunions treated by autologous bone grafting and compression plating. Ann Surg Innov Res. 2009;3:5.

Faldini C, Pagkrati S, Nanni M, et al. Aseptic forearm nonunions treated by plate and opposite fibular autograft strut. Clin Orthop Relat Res. 2009;467(8):2125–34.

Richard MJ, Ruch DS, Aldridge III JM. Malunions and nonunions of the forearm. Hand Clin. 2007;23(2):235–43.

Wrist Arthroscopy

17

Doug A. Campbell

Indications

- To perform an internal examination or treatment in the radiocarpal and/or midcarpal joints.
- There are three categories of indications for wrist arthroscopy:
  - Diagnostic – where the preoperative diagnosis is uncertain
  - Staging – where the diagnosis is known but the stage of disease is not
  - Therapeutic – where a procedure is performed arthroscopically
- Examples of each category are:
  - Diagnostic – causes of wrist pain, confirmation of imaging uncertainties
  - Staging – osteoarthritis, decision-making before proximal row carpectomy
  - Therapeutic – ganglion excision, synovectomy, radial styloidectomy, arthroscopically assisted reduction of scaphoid and distal radius fractures

Preoperative Planning

- Radiographic assessment of the wrist will reveal if there is any unusual carpal anatomy or positioning which could confuse the surgeon on insertion of the arthroscope.

D.A. Campbell
Department of Trauma and Orthopaedic Surgery,
Leeds Teaching Hospitals NHS Trust, Leeds, UK
e-mail: doug.campbell@leedsth.nhs.uk

- A preoperative active dynamic fluoroscopy before anesthesia can be helpful in detailing carpal movements and the source of any clicks/clunks.
- A preoperative examination of the wrist under anesthesia can be helpful in assessing true range of passive movement and stability.

Operative Procedure

- Inform patient of possible complications of:
  - Wound infection (1%)
  - Scar tenderness (temporary)
  - Division of extensor tendon (<1%)
  - Stiffness
  - Bleeding

Anesthesia

- Regional anesthesia is preferred to general anesthesia so that the patient can witness the findings and have them explained to them by the operating surgeon.

Equipment

- A 2.4-mm or 2.7-mm short-barreled wrist arthroscope
- Camera
- Fiber-optic cable
- Light source
- TV camera
- Recording equipment for still photographs and video

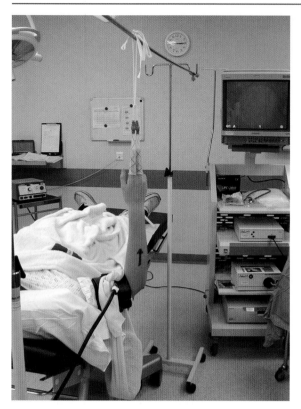

Fig. 17.1 Chinese finger traps attached to index and middle fingers, with limb suspended on a horizontal pole. Humerus parallel to floor. Upper arm tourniquet in place. TV screen placed at patient's feet for viewing by both surgeon and patient

Setup

- Some surgeons prefer to use a specially designed sterile arthroscopic tower which will control the hand/wrist by means of finger traps. The position of the limb can be altered during surgery, and traction can be used if indicated.
- Other surgeons prefer to use Chinese finger traps placed on the index and middle fingers and suspended from a pole between two drip stands (Fig. 17.1). This setup allows the additional use of a mini-C-arm if radiological images are required for the procedure.
- The surgeon will position himself/herself beside the patient's head so that they have access to the dorsal surface of the wrist.
- The TV screen is best placed at the patient's feet so that the surgeon (and patient, if regional anesthetic is used) can see clearly (Fig. 17.1).

Patient Positioning

- Supine.
- Position the upper limb with the humerus parallel to the floor.

Draping and Surgical Approach

- Above elbow tourniquet cuff.
- Sterile drape wrapped around midforearm to occlude upper limb proximal to this level (Fig. 17.2a).
- Sterile drape wrapped around Chinese finger traps if sterile arthroscopic tower not used (Fig. 17.2b).
- Knowledge of surface anatomy is absolutely critical to ensure safe entry of the arthroscope into the joint.
- The important surgical landmarks (Fig. 17.3a) are:
  - Radial styloid
  - Ulnar styloid
  - Lister's tubercle
  - Dorsal rim of distal radius
  - Capitolunate joint
- Two standard portals are used in the radiocarpal joint:
  - The III/IV portal between the III and IV extensor compartments
  - The 6R portal on the radial side of the VI compartment
- One portal is usually used in the midcarpal joint at the level of the capitolunate joint (MC portal).

Radiocarpal Joint Entry

- The dorsal skin of the wrist is stabilized by the surgeon's nondominant thumb. Firm pressure just proximal to the portal will push adjacent extensor tendons out of the way.
- A white needle is inserted into the radiocarpal joint through the III/IV portal area, and sterile saline is injected into the joint (Fig. 17.3b). The contour of the wrist is observed for changes during instillation of approximately 10 mL of sterile fluid.
- A No. 15 blade is inserted into the wrist in the dip just distal to the dorsal rim of the distal radius, approximately 1 cm distal to Lister's tubercle (Fig. 17.4a). The blade must be inserted deep enough to penetrate the joint.

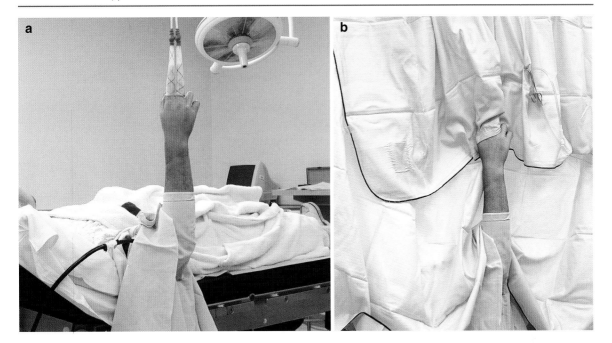

Fig. 17.2 (**a**) Forearm drape in place, (**b**) Upper limb drapes in place

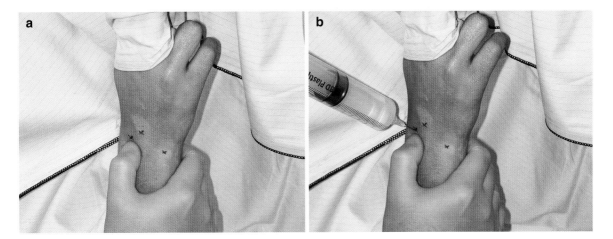

Fig. 17.3 (**a**) Surface landmarks of III/IV, 6R, and MC portals. (**b**) A white needle is inserted into the radiocarpal joint through the III/IV portal

- Without removing his/her thumb, the surgeon then passes a straight small artery forceps through the incision to dilate the portal (Fig. 17.4b).
- The blunt trochar and introducer are inserted into the radiocarpal joint (Fig. 17.4c). If any resistance is experienced, the surgeon must not push hard to insert the trochar. A sharp trochar must never be used.

- The trochar is removed from its sleeve, and a sterile saline irrigation system attached. The irrigation is turned on to force air bubbles out of the joint.
- The arthroscope is inserted through the introducer (Fig. 17.4d), and a complete examination of the joint is performed (see later).
- A second portal is usually used to allow a blunt probe to assist in examination. The 6R portal on the radial

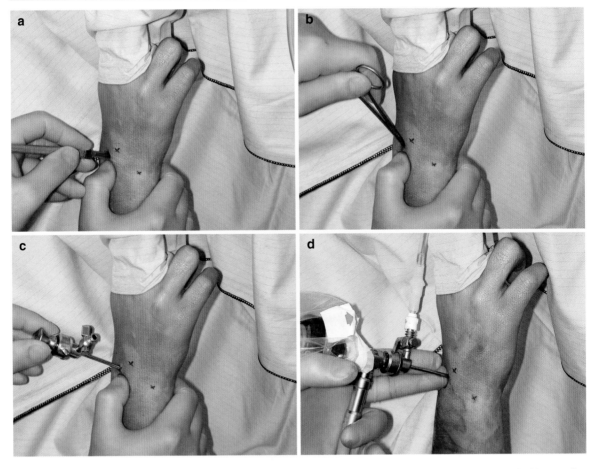

Fig. 17.4 (**a**) A No. 15 blade is inserted into the radiocarpal joint while the surrounding skin and deeper structures are stabilized. (**b**) Straight artery forceps are passed into the radiocarpal joint to establish the portal. (**c**) An introducer with blunt trochar is passed into the radiocarpal joint. (**d**) The arthroscope is passed through the introducer and into the radiocarpal joint

side of the extensor carpi ulnaris (ECU) tendon is created in a similar manner to the III/IV portal.

Midcarpal Joint Entry

- The entry point is found in the palpable dip just distal to the III/IV portal but more towards the midline of the wrist.
- The angle of entry of the needle into the midcarpal joint is much steeper than into the radiocarpal joint (Fig. 17.5).
- A similar sequence of events to that described above is employed in inserting the arthroscope.
- A thorough examination of the joint is performed (see later).

Radiocarpal Joint Examination

- A thorough and repeatable journey must be undertaken.
- Accurate knowledge of the anatomy is mandatory.
- Begin by identifying a localizing structure, most usually the scapholunate junction.
- This is done by slowly withdrawing the arthroscope until the two bones of the scaphoid (radially) and lunate (ulnarly) are visualized superiorly. The junction between these two bones forms a "dip" often likened to the natal cleft (Fig. 17.6).
- Once the position of the arthroscope is confirmed, begin by passing the scope radially to visualize the scaphoid and its synovial reflection superiorly and the radial styloid inferiorly.

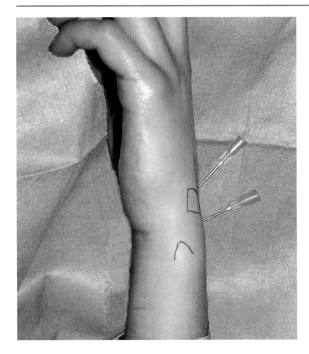

Fig. 17.5 The angle of entry is much steeper into the midcarpal joint

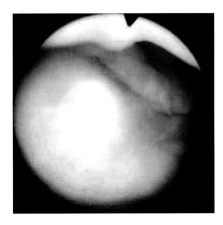

Fig. 17.6 The scapholunate joint

- Document the findings at each stage in this journey.
- Next, move the arthroscope in an ulnar direction, examining the scaphoid fossa of the distal radius inferiorly with the proximal pole of the scaphoid superiorly, then passing the scapholunate junction superiorly and the interfossa ridge of the distal radius inferiorly.
- Now, examine the lunate superiorly and the lunate fossa of the distal radius inferiorly. Finally, move into the ulnar side of the radiocarpal joint.

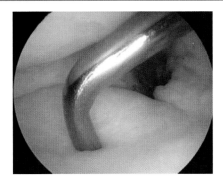

Fig. 17.7 The trampoline test – note the fovea in the background

- Here, examine the triangular fibrocartilage inferiorly together with assessing the integrity of its attachments to the sigmoid notch of the distal radius and the dorsal and palmar peripheries with a blunt hook inserted through the 6R portal.
- Assess the tension in the TFCC by "bouncing" the blunt hook against it and looking for elastic recoil (the "trampoline" test) (Fig. 17.7).
- Do not be confused by the fovea – a dorsal ulnar pit with proliferative synovium often visible within. This is not a dorsal detachment.
- It is possible to visualize the undersurface of the pisiform in some individuals, and an attempt should be made to do this. Pass the arthroscope in a palmar ulnar direction around the edge of the triquetrum to see if this possible.
- Once the inspection and probing of each structure is complete, remove the arthroscope and prepare to examine the midcarpal joint.

Midcarpal Joint Examination

- The point of orientation is the capitate head lying superiorly and ulnarly and the scapholunate junction lying inferiorly.
- Move the arthroscope in a radial direction to examine the scaphocapitate joint. At its most superior extreme, the trapezium can usually be visualized together with the scaphotrapeziotrapezoid (STT) joint surfaces.
- On returning to the point of entry, note the relationship between the scaphoid and lunate. Is there evidence of a step-off here or fibrillation of the edge of

one or both bones, suggesting abnormal movement? Attempt to open this junction with the arthroscope to see if a gap can be visualized.

- Now, move the arthroscope in an ulnar direction to examine the lunotriquetral joint inferiorly (again performing the examination noted above for the scapholunate joint) while also noting the condition of the surface of the capitate superiorly.
- Further ulnar movement of the arthroscope will allow visualization of the capitohamate joint and, finally, the bare dorsal surface of the hamate.

Documentation

- It is critical to accurately record each stage of the arthroscopic journey. It will not be possible to remember specific details when reviewing the patient weeks or months later.
- It is also important to record which portals were used, the clarity or ease of visualization of structures, and any abnormalities in preoperative examination or arthroscopic assessment.
- It is recommended to reexamine the wrist clinically some weeks after diagnostic arthroscopy, bearing in mind the arthroscopic findings. These findings may not always be relevant to the presenting complaint.

Closure

- Steristrips alone are all that is necessary. Sutures are not required.
- A bulky, but not tight, wool and crepe bandage is recommended to be worn for 7 days after surgery.

Postoperative Rehabilitation

- Return to preoperative activities will depend on what is found or performed during arthroscopic examination.
- In the simplest of cases, where a diagnostic examination alone is performed, patients can return to full activities as soon as their wounds have healed and their comfort allows. This is usually around 7–10 days after arthroscopy.

Follow-up

- It is recommended that an outpatient review is carried out with the findings of diagnostic arthroscopy available. This is usually done around 2–4 weeks after surgery. It is essential to check the integrity of the finger and thumb extensors at this visit since inadvertent division during arthroscopy has been reported.
- The patient can be discharged when no further treatments are planned or definitive treatment has supervened.

Further Reading

Siparsky PN, Kocher MS. Current concepts in pediatric and adolescent arthroscopy. Arthroscopy. 2009;25(12): 1453–69.
Chloros GD, Wiesler ER, Poehling GG. Current concepts in wrist arthroscopy. Arthroscopy. 2008;24(3):343–54.
Puhaindran ME, Yam AK, Chin AY, et al. Wrist arthroscopy: beware the novice. J Hand Surg Eur Vol. 2009;34(4): 540–2.

Wrist Arthrodesis

Robert Farnell

Indications

- Painful wrist (radiocarpal and/or midcarpal) joint where reconstructive surgical options are not possible. Typical conditions treated with a wrist arthrodesis are:
  - Osteoarthritis (from SLAC, SNAC, post wrist fracture, Kienbock's disease)
  - Rheumatoid arthritis
  - Unsuccessful total joint arthroplasty
  - Spastic hemiplegia with wrist flexion
  - Painful instability

Contraindications

- Active infection.
- CRPS.
- Poor finger function.
- Poor skin quality.

Preoperative Planning

Clinical Assessment

- Painful radiocarpal joint movement which is limiting function and not controlled by nonoperative measures.

R. Farnell
Department of Trauma and Orthopaedic Surgery,
Leeds Teaching Hospitals NHS Trust,
Leeds, UK
e-mail: robert.farnell@leedsth.nhs.uk

Radiological Assessment

- Posteroanterior and lateral wrist X-ray within 3 months of the surgical date (Fig. 18.1).

Preoperative Consent

- Fully explain the procedure and that there will be a permanent visible scar. The wrist will be in a plaster cast for 6 weeks postoperatively. In the first few days, it is likely to be painful, and regular analgesia will be required.
- Discuss the postoperative risks, including wound infection, surgical scarring, bleeding, and injury to the extensor tendons. There is a risk of the arthrodesis not uniting, resulting in persistent pain and further surgery. Metalwork removal may be necessary.
- Mark the limb.

Operative Treatment

Anesthesia

- Regional (brachial plexus) nerve block or general anesthesia.
- At induction, administer prophylactic antibiotic as per local hospital protocol (e.g., cephalosporin).

Equipment

- Image intensifier or fluoroscan.
- Radiolucent arm table attached to the operating table.

Fig. 18.1 Preoperative
X-ray – in this case, a
scapholunate advanced
collapse (*SLAC*) wrist

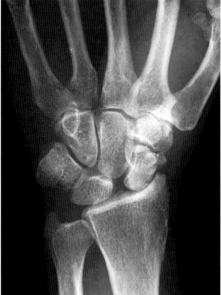
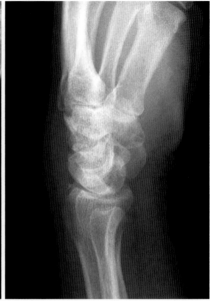

Fig. 18.2 The Synthes® wrist
arthrodesis set

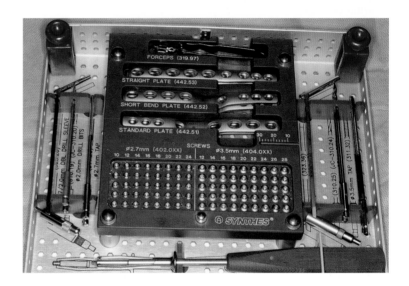

- Complete set of wrist arthrodesis implants with instrumentation and power drills (Fig. 18.2).
- Synthetic bone graft (or allograft).
- Osteotomes.

Patient Positioning

- Patient supine, with the arm lying on the arm table which is attached to the operating table.
- Fit a high arm pneumatic tourniquet.

Draping and Surgical Approach

- Prepare the skin of the hand, forearm, and upper arm to the level of the tourniquet using the usual antiseptic solutions (e.g., aqueous povidone-iodine).
- Use an upper extremity arm drape, which also covers the arm table (Fig. 18.3a).
- Exsanguinate the arm with a sterile Esmarch's bandage (Fig. 18.3b).

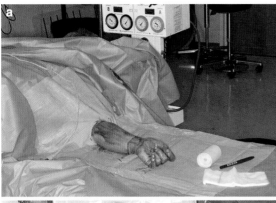

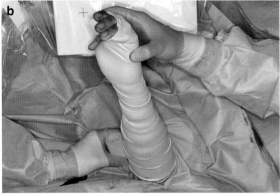

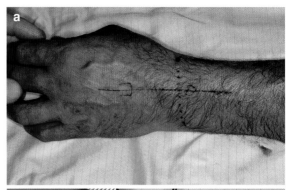

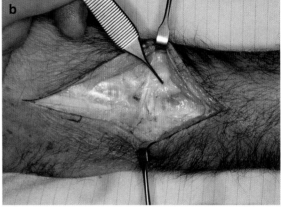

Fig. 18.3 (**a**) Preparation with a pneumatic tourniquet, upper limb exclusion drape, and bipolar diathermy. (**b**) Exsanguination with a sterile Esmarch's bandage

Fig. 18.4 (**a**) Skin incision. Lister's tubercle and the middle CMCJ are shown. The *dotted line* shows the radiocarpal joint. (**b**) The extensor retinaculum is shown by the forceps tips. The EPL tendon is beneath the forceps, lying immediately ulnar to Lister's tubercle

- Use a dorsal midline incision beginning 6 cm proximal to Lister's tubercle to the middle of the middle metacarpal (Fig. 18.4a).
- Divide and ligate any large subcutaneous veins until the layer of the extensor retinaculum and forearm fascia is reached.
- Identify the extensor pollicis longus tendon (EPL) as it passes obliquely around Lister's tubercle distal to the extensor retinaculum (Fig. 18.4b).
- Open up the compartment in which EPL lies (the third extensor compartment) (Fig. 18.5a). Retract the EPL tendon (Fig. 18.5b).
- Subperiosteally elevate the soft tissue from the distal radius in a radial and ulnar direction (Fig. 18.6).

Procedure

- Continue elevating the soft tissues and extrinsic wrist ligaments to expose the carpal bones and the

radiocarpal, midcarpal, and third carpometacarpal (CMC) joints (Fig. 18.7a).
- Place the wrist arthrodesis plate in the position that it is to be used – this is along the long axis of the radius and middle metacarpal bones. Remove the prominent Lister's tubercle and dorsal distal radius with an osteotome so that the plate lies comfortably on the bone surfaces. Keep this bone for use as a graft (Fig. 18.7b).
- Replace the arthrodesis plate and drill one hole in the distal radius and one hole in the middle metacarpal (Fig. 18.8). These drill holes ensure that when the plate is finally applied, there is no loss of radial/carpal height, thereby preventing an effective ulnar lengthening (abutment), which can occur after removal of the articular surfaces. If there is a significant degree of radial or ulnar deformity, the alignment can be fine-tuned later. 2.7-mm screws

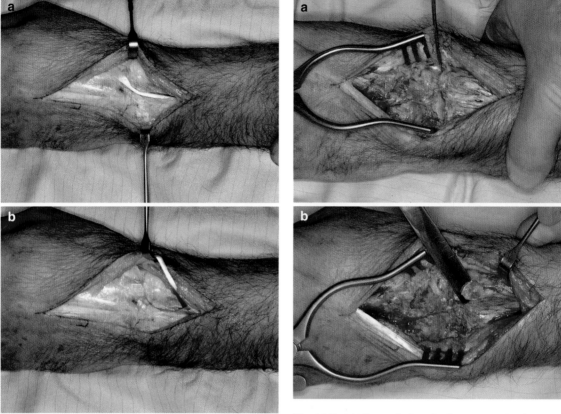

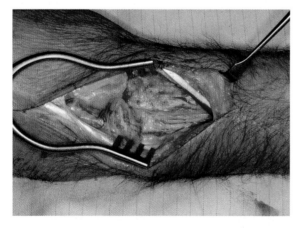

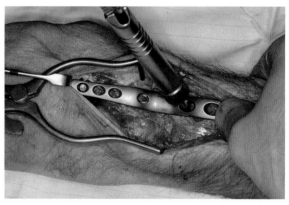

Fig. 18.5 (**a**) The third extensor compartment is opened to show the EPL tendon. (**b**) The EPL tendon is elevated from its bed

Fig. 18.7 (**a**) The extrinsic wrist ligaments and soft tissue are elevated off the carpal bones to reveal the radiocarpal, midcarpal, and middle CMC joints. The bone lever has been placed in the radiocarpal joint for identification purposes. (**b**) Lister's tubercle and any prominent distal radius are removed with an osteotome, and the bone saved for use as bone graft

Fig. 18.6 The distal radius has been exposed by subperiosteally elevating the soft tissues

Fig. 18.8 The arthrodesis plate is applied and holes drilled into the distal radius and middle metacarpal so that no loss in carpal height occurs. Here the length of the screw is being measured

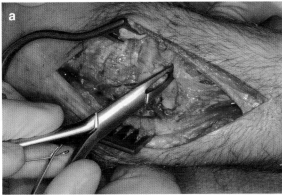

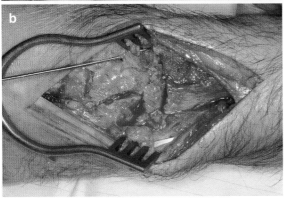

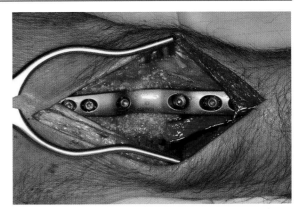

Fig. 18.10 The arthrodesis plate has been applied for definitive fixation. Synthetic bone graft has been inserted into the joint surfaces

Fig. 18.9 (**a**) The articular surfaces are prepared removing the cartilage down to healthy cancellous bone. (**b**) Complete preparation of the articular surfaces has been achieved. A temporary K-wire was inserted into the scaphoid to permit good access to the proximal pole surface. The middle CMCJ has also been prepared

Closure

- Repair the extensor retinaculum with 4/0 Vicryl. Leave the extensor pollicis longus tendon superficial to the retinaculum to protect it from rupture (Fig. 18.11a).
- Skin closure with 3/0 subcuticular Prolene (Fig. 18.11b).
- Petroleum jelly gauze, dressing gauze, Velband, and volar plaster of Paris slab (Fig. 18.12).
- Release the tourniquet.

Postoperative Rehabilitation

- Overnight admission and elevation in a Bradford sling.
- Opiate analgesia is often required in the first 24 h.
- Administer regular analgesia for 48–72 h. An opiate and paracetamol combination is usually sufficient.

Outpatient Follow-up

- 2 weeks: Suture removal and apply a new lightweight wrist cast.
- 6 weeks: Remove the cast and X-ray. If this looks satisfactory, begin mobilization (Fig. 18.13).
- Follow up until there is radiological confirmation of union and symptom resolution.

are used for the metacarpal; 3.5-mm screws, in the distal radius.

- Remove the articular cartilage and subchondral bone to expose cancellous bone in the distal radius, scaphoid, lunate, triquetrum, capitate, and hamate (Fig. 18.9a). There is debate about whether to arthrodese the middle carpometacarpal joint (CMCJ). If it is decided to include this joint, it will also need to be prepared in a similar manner (Fig. 18.9b).
- Apply the arthrodesis plate using the previously drilled holes. Add further screws so that there are three in the distal radius and middle metacarpal and one in the capitate. Use the image intensifier to ensure that the screws are not too long, risking tendon injury in the carpal tunnel and palm.
- Insert the bone removed from the distal radius into the joint surfaces and augment this with synthetic graft/processed bone if required (Fig. 18.10).

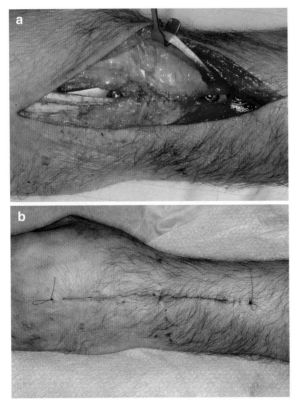

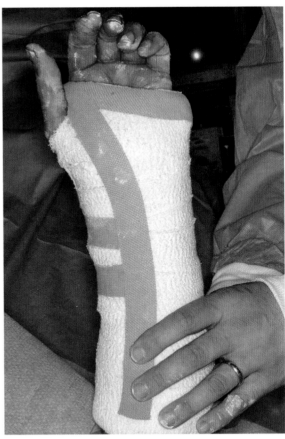

Fig. 18.11 (**a**) The extensor retinaculum is closed with 4/0 Vicryl, leaving the EPL tendon superficial. (**b**) Skin closure with a subcuticular Prolene suture

Fig. 18.12 Dressing with volar plaster of Paris slab, leaving the MCP joints free to allow finger mobilization

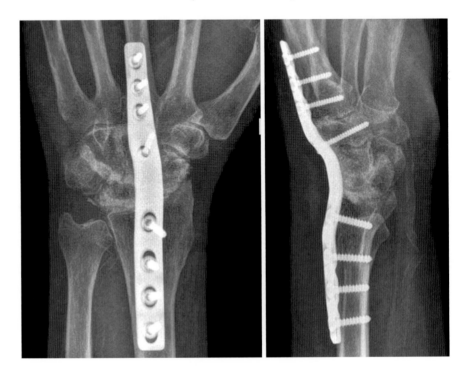

Fig. 18.13 A 6-week postoperative X-ray

Tips

- Another valid surgical alternative are the limited or partial wrist fusions. With those operations, the functional range of motion is preserved compared with the total fusion as the intercarpal joints remained intact. The load is transferred to the uninjured wrist site in such a way to protect the injured row from further degeneration – arthritis.
- The surgeon must consider that healthy joints are not fused. The volume of the bones that are going to be fused must be preserved. The internal fixation involves only the bones incorporated in the fusion.
- Partial wrist fusions were classified as radiocarpal, midcarpal, and intercarpal and are advised to be performed by expert surgeons in the field.

Implant Removal

- Not usually required unless the middle CMCJ has not been fused.

Further Reading

Anderson MC, Adams BD. Total wrist arthroplasty. Hand Clin. 2005;21(4):621–30.

Weiss AP. Osteoarthritis of the wrist. Instr Course Lect. 2004;53:31–40.

Cavaliere CM, Chung KC. A systematic review of total wrist arthroplasty compared with total wrist arthrodesis for rheumatoid arthritis. Plast Reconstr Surg. 2008;122(3):813–25.

Watson HK, Weinzweig J, Guidera PM, et al. One thousand intercarpal arthrodeses. J Hand Surg Br. 1999;24(3): 307–15.

Scaphoid Nonunion

19

Doug A. Campbell

Indications

- Nonunion of a scaphoid fracture.
- This description relates to a palmar approach for the more common nonunions in the scaphoid waist.

Preoperative Planning

Clinical Assessment

- Document range of motion, grip strength and describe painful activities.
- Consider whether grafting is indicated based on absence of secondary degenerative disease.
- Discuss the possible complications of:
  - Wound infection
  - Stiffness
  - Persistent nonunion
  - Bleeding
  - Scar tenderness

Operative Procedure

Surface Markings

- Identify subcutaneous course of flexor carpi radialis tendon (FCR).

- Place incision along distal course of FCR as it passes radially around the scaphoid tubercle (Fig. 19.1).

Anesthesia

- General or regional anesthetic is essential.
- A single dose of intravenous antibiotic prophylaxis is given before incision.

Equipment

- A standard set of fine surgical instruments, including scissors, fine-toothed forceps, self-retaining retractor, handheld small retractor, and needle holders.
- A suitable implant for scaphoid fixation (such as a headless screw).
- Equipment for creating and harvesting a small bone graft.
- An image intensifier.

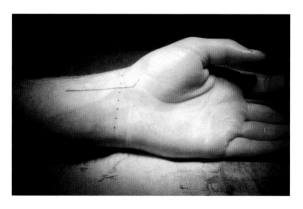

Fig. 19.1 Surface markings of skin incision

D.A. Campbell
Department of Trauma and Orthopaedic Surgery,
Leeds Teaching Hospitals NHS Trust,
Leeds, UK
e-mail: doug.campbell@leedsth.nhs.uk

P.V. Giannoudis (ed.), *Practical Procedures in Elective Orthopaedic Surgery*,
DOI 10.1007/978-0-85729-820-1_19, © Springer-Verlag London Limited 2012

Fig. 19.2 Preparation and draping of the upper limb

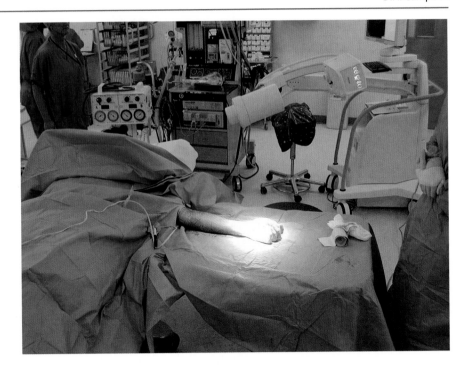

Patient Positioning

- Supine.
- Affected arm on hand table.
- Ensure patient comfort before inflating tourniquet if under regional anesthesia.

Draping and Surgical Approach

- Above elbow tourniquet cuff.
- Sterile drape wrapped around upper arm at level of tourniquet cuff (Fig. 19.2).
- Arm exsanguinated to level of tourniquet cuff.

Surgical Procedure

- Incision along line of distal course of FCR, curved radially around scaphoid tubercle.
- Identify FCR and release it from its sheath.
- Open the deep layer of the FCR sheath and carefully dissect to the radial side of the tendon of flexor pollicis longus (FPL).

- Identify the scaphoid tubercle and dissect sharply around it and proximally to enter the radioscaphoid joint.
- Pass a blunt elevator into the radioscaphoid joint to identify the nonunion in the scaphoid (Fig. 19.3a).
- Resect the area of nonunion with sharp osteotomes to create two opposing flat surfaces.
- Resect sufficient bone until healthy cancellous surface is visible.
- Measure the distance between the flat cancellous surfaces using small osteotomes (Fig. 19.3b).
- Return to the proximal aspect of the wound to harvest a bone graft from the distal radius.
- Carefully expose the fascia over pronator quadratus (PQ) (Fig. 19.4).
- Incise the fascia to reveal the underlying muscle.
- Pass a blunt elevator deep to the PQ muscle to create an extra periosteal plane (Fig. 19.5a, b).
- Should a vascularised bone graft be indicated, seek and identify the transverse volar radial carpal artery – which passes transversely from the radial artery to the anterior interosseous artery and lies just distal to the distal edge of PQ (Fig. 19.6a).

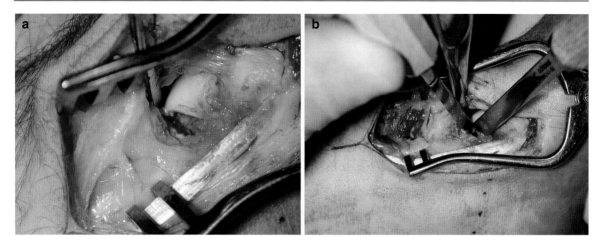

Fig. 19.3 (**a**) Blunt elevator in radioscaphoid joint. (**b**) Measure the defect size

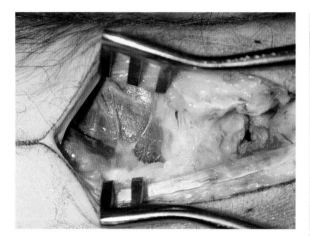

Fig. 19.4 Pronator quadratus (PQ)

- Carefully elevate the volar radial carpal artery from the underlying periosteum, taking care to leave sufficient soft tissue around the pedicle (for venous drainage) (Fig. 19.6b).
- Using bipolar diathermy, divide the pedicle as it crosses the ulnar margin of the distal radius.
- Plan the bone graft harvest from the volar surface of the distal radius, cutting the thickest area of bone (the most proximal) first to reduce the risk of corticocancellous separation.
- Place a hypodermic needle in the radiocarpal joint to prevent inadvertent bone graft harvest from the articular surface (Fig. 19.7).

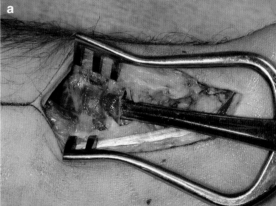

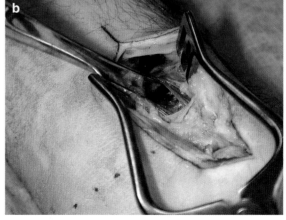

Fig. 19.5 (**a**) Blunt elevator is passed deep to PQ. (**b**) Extra periosteal dissection reveals surface vessels

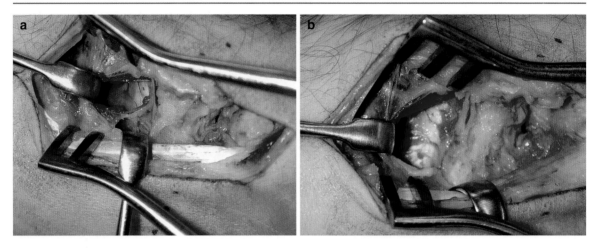

Fig. 19.6 (**a**) The volar radial carpal artery. (**b**) Mobilize the pedicle

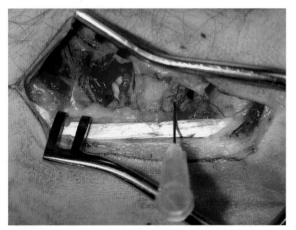

Fig. 19.7 Mark the radiocarpal joint with a needle

- Raise the bone graft on its pedicle and free the pedicle to the pivot point (origin from radial artery) (Fig. 19.8a).
- Rotate the graft around, taking care not to twist the pedicle, and place in previously created defect in scaphoid (Fig. 19.8b).

Screw Insertion

- To identify the correct entry point for the scaphoid screw, remove the overhanging ridge of the trapezium with a sharp osteotome (Fig. 19.9).

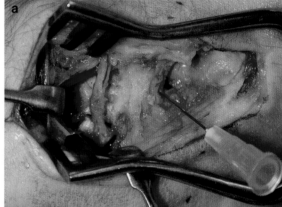

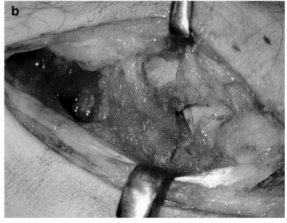

Fig. 19.8 (**a**) Raise and mobilize the graft and its pedicle. (**b**) Place the graft in the defect

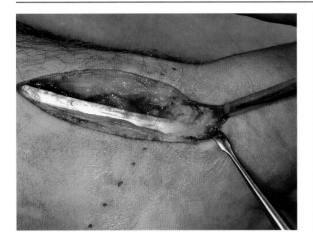

Fig. 19.9 Expose the entry point for the implant

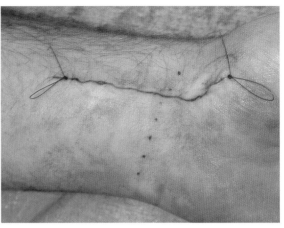

Fig. 19.11 Skin closure

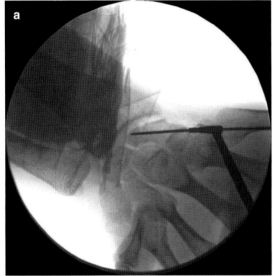

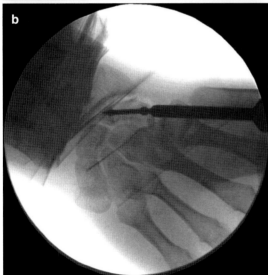

Fig. 19.10 (a) Insert the guide wire. (b) Insert the implant

- Pass a threaded guide wire under image intensifier control, such that it crosses both poles of the scaphoid and the interposed bone graft (Fig. 19.10a).
- Ensure the guide wire passes along the long axis of the scaphoid.
- Check the position of the guide wire from different angles using the image intensifier.
- Insert the screw using interfragmentary compression to stabilize the construct (Fig. 19.10b).
- On some occasions, a parallel K-wire is inserted to prevent rotational displacement of the proximal pole as the screw is tightened.

Closure

- Using a cannulated screw negates the need to open and divide the palmar extrinsic ligaments. Their repair is therefore unnecessary.
- Carefully close the deep layer of the FCR sheath using absorbable 4/0 sutures. Be careful not to damage the graft pedicle.
- Close the skin with interrupted sutures or continuous subcuticular sutures (Fig. 19.11). Great care must be taken to prevent overlapping the skin edges on closure since this will lead to a tender and hypertrophic scar.
- Apply a bulky, padded bandage with a plaster of Paris half splint extending around the thumb for comfort (Fig. 19.12).

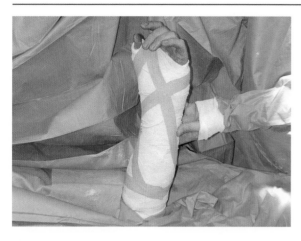

Fig. 19.12 Bulky dressing with plaster of Paris splint

Postoperative Rehabilitation

- Remove sutures, if nonabsorbable, at 10–12 days.
- Apply a full scaphoid cast, to be worn until 6 weeks after surgery.

Outpatient Review

- Wound check and suture removal/plaster cast application at 10–12 days.
- X-rays at 10–12 days (to confirm implant position), 6 weeks (to assess union), and 3 months (to, hopefully, confirm union).
- The patient can be discharged once radiological union has occurred.
- The implant does not need to be removed.

Further Reading

Kawamura K, Chung KC. Treatment of scaphoid fractures and nonunions. J Hand Surg Am. 2008;33(6):988–97.

Steinmann SP, Adams JE. Scaphoid fractures and nonunions: diagnosis and treatment. J Orthop Sci. 2006;11(4):424–31.

Trumble TE, Salas P, Barthel T, et al. Management of scaphoid nonunions. J Am Acad Orthop Surg. 2003;11(6):380–91.

Payatakes A, Sotereanos DG. Pedicled vascularized bone grafts for scaphoid and lunate reconstruction. J Am Acad Orthop Surg. 2009;17(12):744–55.

Trapezectomy

20

Robert Farnell

Indications

- Symptomatic osteoarthritis carpometacarpal (CMC) thumb joint not controlled by nonoperative treatment.
- Symptomatic pantrapezial thumb osteoarthritis.

Contraindications

- Active infection.
- CRPS.

Preoperative Planning

Clinical Assessment

- Ensure the symptoms are arising from the CMC joint. This is confirmed by reproducing the symptoms by stressing the CMCJ (a positive ballottement or grind test).
- Assess the degree of thumb metacarpophalangeal joint (CMCJ) hyperextension. If this is greater than 30°, consider performing volar plate advancement at the same time.

Radiological Assessment

- Posteroanterior and lateral (Fig. 20.1) thumb X-ray within 3 months of the operation date.

Preoperative Consent

- The indication for surgery is pain. Explain that it can take up to 1 year for the pain to completely resolve.

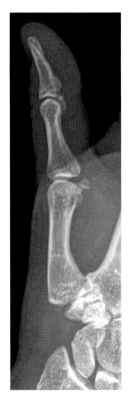

Fig. 20.1 Preoperative lateral X-ray showing carpometacarpal osteoarthritis

R. Farnell
Department of Trauma and Orthopaedic Surgery,
Leeds Teaching Hospitals NHS Trust,
Leeds, UK
e-mail: robert.farnell@leedsth.nhs.uk

P.V. Giannoudis (ed.), *Practical Procedures in Elective Orthopaedic Surgery*,
DOI 10.1007/978-0-85729-820-1_20, © Springer-Verlag London Limited 2012

- Discuss the risks of surgery – infection (1%), visible surgical scar, injury to the radial sensory nerve, radial artery injury, and bleeding or thumb stiffness. The patient may be aware that their thumb is a slightly shorter and "floppier" thumb. Their maximal thumb pinch will be reduced compared to a normal individual, but as the pain is reduced their pinch grip will be greater than it currently is.
- Mark the limb.

Operative Treatment

Anesthesia

- Regional (brachial plexus) nerve block or general anesthesia.
- Prophylactic antibiotics are not routinely given, but check your local hospital protocol.

Equipment

- Radiolucent arm table attached to the operating table.
- Fine bone rongeurs.
- Small osteotomes.
- Bipolar diathermy.

Patient Positioning

- Patient supine with the arm lying on an arm table attached to the operating table.
- Fit a high arm pneumatic tourniquet.

Draping and Surgical Approach

- Prepare the skin of the hand, forearm, and upper arm to the level of the tourniquet using the usual antiseptic solution (e.g., aqueous povidone iodine).
- Use an upper extremity drape which also covers the arm table.
- Mark the proposed skin incision with a pen (Fig. 20.2).
- Exsanguinate the arm with a sterile Esmarch bandage.

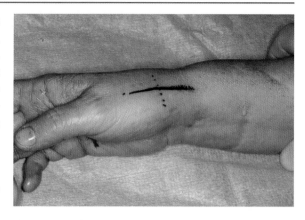

Fig. 20.2 Skin marking for incision. The CMCJ is indicated by the *dotted line*

Procedure

- Use a dorsal midline incision centered on the thumb CMCJ (Fig. 20.3a).
- Identify and gently protect branches of the radial sensory nerve. These do not tolerate retraction or injury and can result in painful neuroma formation (Fig. 20.3b).
- Approach the CMCJ through a longitudinal incision on the ulnar side of the first extensor compartment tendons (abductor pollicis longus and extensor pollicis brevis tendons).
- Identify the deep branch of the radial artery as it crosses the trapezium and distal scaphoid obliquely (Fig. 20.4a). Gently mobilize the artery, which usually requires dividing two to three small deep arterial branches with the bipolar diathermy. Protect the artery with a small retractor (Fig. 20.4b).
- Incise the CMCJ capsule and subperiosteally elevate it off the metacarpal base and trapezium (Fig. 20.5a).
- Incise the capsule of the STT joint and ensure that the bone that you are planning to remove is the trapezium (there are reports of surgeons inadvertently removing the scaphoid bone). Identification is made by visualizing the CMC joint, which is saddle-shaped, and the distal pole of the scaphoid at the STT joint, which is convex (Fig. 20.5b).
- Elevate as much periosteum off the trapezium as possible as this makes removal easier.
- Remove the trapezium bone, which in this case is done piecemeal. An osteotome is used to break the

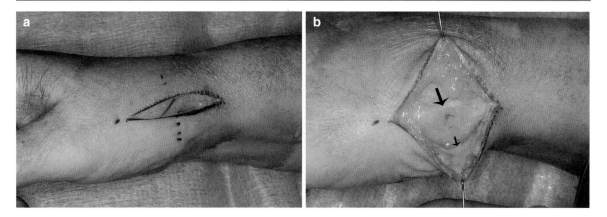

Fig. 20.3 (**a**) Skin incision. (**b**) The sensory branch of the radial nerve (*small arrow*) and EPB tendon (*large arrow*)

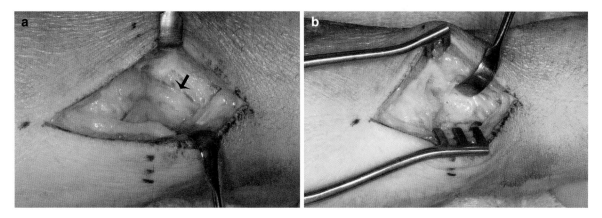

Fig. 20.4 (**a**) Deeper dissection. The EPB tendon has been retracted radially and deep branch of the radial artery can be seen crossing the operative field (*arrow*). (**b**) The radial artery has been mobilized and gently retracted proximally

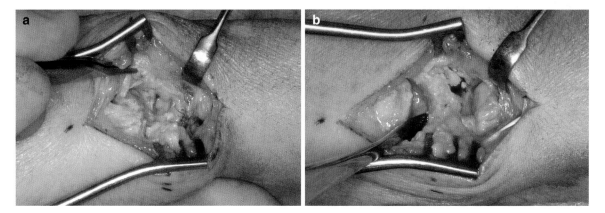

Fig. 20.5 (**a**) Subperisosteal elevation of the capsule to expose the trapezium bone. (**b**) The trapezium is identified. The bone lever has been placed in the CMCJ, which is saddle-shaped. Proximal to this, the convex distal pole of the scaphoid can be seen (there is some cartilage loss here in this case indicating pantrapezial joint arthritis despite an apparently normal joint on X-ray)

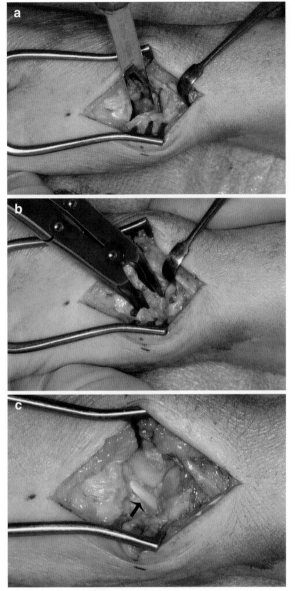

Fig. 20.6 (**a**) An osteotome is used to break the trapezium into two pieces. (**b**) The trapezium is removed piecemeal. (**c**) The trapezium has been removed and the FCR tendon (*arrow*) can be seen at the base of the wound. The articular surfaces of the trapezoid and distal pole of scaphoid can also be clearly seen

trapezium in two (Fig. 20.6a), and the bone removed using bone rongeurs (Fig. 20.6b). As the trapezium is removed, be careful to identify and protect the flexor carpi radialis (FCR) tendon as it grooves the deep surface of the trapezium passing from palmar to dorsal (Fig. 20.6c).

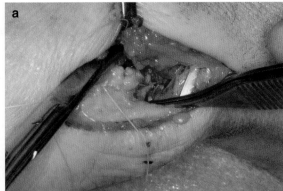

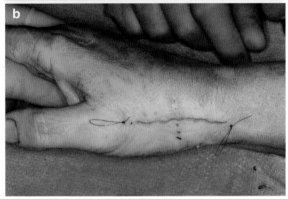

Fig. 20.7 (**a**) Closure of the capsule with 4/0 Vicryl. (**b**) Skin closure with a continuous subcuticular 3/0 Prolene suture

• Ensure any osteophytes between the thumb and index metacarpals are removed.

Closure

• Capsule – 4/0 Vicryl (Fig. 20.7a).
• Skin – 3/0 subcuticular Prolene (Fig. 20.7b).
• Dressing – petroleum jelly gauze, dressing gauze, velband, and a crepe bandage with a volar plaster of Paris slab, including the thumb (Fig. 20.8a, b).
• Release the tourniquet.

Postoperative Rehabilitation

• Elevate in a sling and encourage finger mobilization.
• Prescribe regular analgesia for 48 h followed by analgesia as required. A codeine and paracetamol

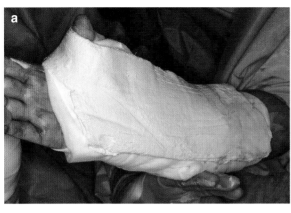
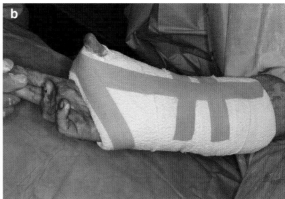

Fig. 20.8 (**a**) A volar plaster of Paris slab is applied which includes the thumb. (**b**) The final dressing

combination and/or nonsteroidal anti-inflammatory medication are usually sufficient.

Outpatients Follow-up

- 2 weeks:
  - Cast and suture removal.
  - Fit a thermoplastic splint to include the thumb which is worn for 4 weeks.

- 3–6 months:
  - Ensure recovery progressing.
  - Warn the patient that improvements often continue for up to 1 year after surgery.

Further Reading

Wright TW, Thompson J, Conrad BP. Loading of the index metacarpal after trapezial and partial versus complete trapezoid resection. J Hand Surg Am. 2006;31(1):58–62.

Carpal Tunnel Release

21

Doug A. Campbell

Indications

- Carpal tunnel syndrome.

Preoperative Planning

Clinical Assessment

- Symptoms
  - Median innervated dysesthesia
  - Nocturnal symptoms
  - Clumsiness – loss of fine touch appreciation (= "tactile blindness")
- Signs
  - Wasting/weakness of abductor pollicis brevis (APB)
  - Normal sensation of skin over thenar eminence
  - Localizing signs at wrist level (positive Tinel's test and/or Phalen's test)

Electrophysiological Assessment

- Not always necessary if clinical symptoms sufficiently clear.
- Likely to reveal conduction delay in median nerve at level of wrist.

D.A. Campbell
Department of Trauma and Orthopaedic Surgery,
Leeds Teaching Hospitals NHS Trust,
Leeds, UK
e-mail: doug.campbell@leedsth.nhs.uk

Differential Diagnoses

- Cervical root entrapment (C6 dermatome).
- Diabetic neuropathy.
- Other causes of neuropathy (e.g., alcohol, neoplasia, nutritional disease, etc.).

Operative Procedure

- Inform of possible complications
  - Wound infection (1%)
  - Scar tenderness

Surface Markings

- Knowledge of surface anatomy is critical to placing incision correctly.
- The important surgical landmarks (Fig. 21.1) are:
  - Proximal limit of carpal tunnel
  - Pisiform
  - Scaphoid tubercle
  - Distal limit of carpal tunnel
  - Hook of hamate
  - Ridge of trapezium
- Make a line along the palm between the third web space and the interthenar depression (Fig. 21.1).
- The skin incision is placed along this line between the proximal and distal limits of the tunnel (Fig. 21.2).

P.V. Giannoudis (ed.), *Practical Procedures in Elective Orthopaedic Surgery*,
DOI 10.1007/978-0-85729-820-1_21, © Springer-Verlag London Limited 2012

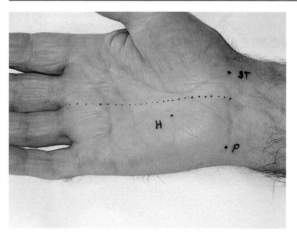

Fig. 21.1 Surface markings of carpal tunnel (*P* pisiform, *H* hamate, *ST* scaphoid tubercle) and from third web space to wrist crease

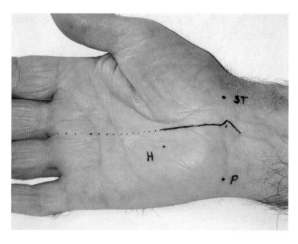

Fig. 21.2 Proposed incision marked on line from third web space between marked limits of carpal tunnel

Anesthesia

- Local anesthetic infiltration is almost always preferred.
- Adrenaline can be added to reduce bleeding and prolong anesthetic efficacy.
- Skin must be infiltrated proximal to wrist crease first (loose skin and less painful) (Fig. 21.3a).
- Skin and subcutaneous tissue SLOWLY infiltrated to beyond surface marking of distal limit of carpal tunnel (Fig. 21.3b).

Equipment

- A standard set of fine surgical instruments including scissors, fine-toothed forceps, self-retaining retractor, handheld small retractor, needle holders

Patient Positioning

- Supine.
- Affected arm on hand table.
- Ensure patient comfort before inflating tourniquet.

Draping and Surgical Approach

- Above elbow tourniquet cuff (Fig. 21.4a).
- Sterile drape wrapped around upper arm at level of tourniquet cuff (Fig. 21.4b).
- Arm exsanguinated to level of tourniquet cuff (Fig. 21.4c).

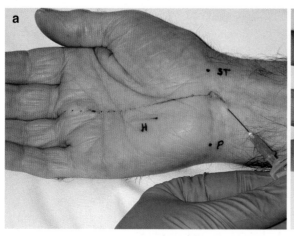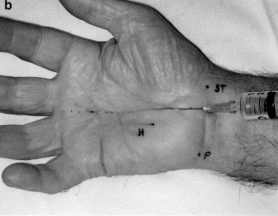

Fig. 21.3 (**a**) Local anesthetic infiltrated into loose skin proximal to wrist flexion crease (**b**) and along line of proposed incision

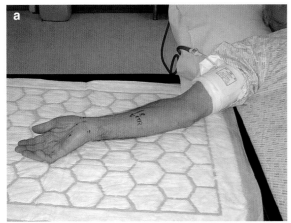

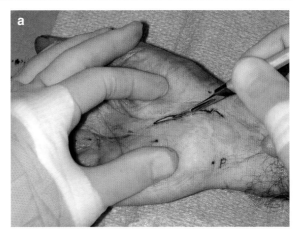

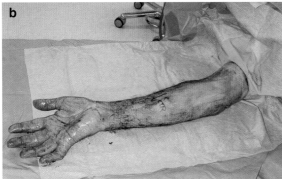

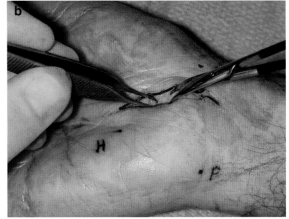

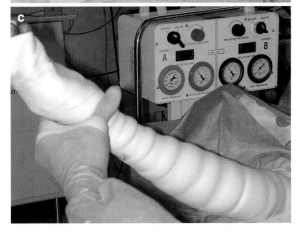

Fig. 21.5 (**a**) Incision is made with knife perpendicular to skin surface. (**b**) Subcutaneous tissues gently spread in search of superficial nerves

Fig. 21.4 (**a**) Application of padded above elbow tourniquet cuff. (**b**) Sterile drape to expose upper limb prepared to level of tourniquet cuff and (**c**) exsanguination to level of tourniquet cuff

Surgical Procedure

- Straight incision in line with third web space between pre-marked proximal and distal limits of carpal tunnel.
- Zigzag or angled extension proximally across wrist crease.
- Ensure knife is perpendicular to skin surface (Fig. 21.5a).

- Carefully separate subcutaneous layer to look for sensory nerve fibers (Fig. 21.5b).
- Once superficial fascia is reached along the entire length of incision, insert self-retaining or handheld retractors (Fig. 21.6a).
- Divide superficial fascia under direct vision to reveal flexor retinaculum (Fig. 21.6b).
- Look out for aberrant motor branches which can pierce the retinaculum from deep to superficial.
- Divide flexor retinaculum using a fresh blade. Do not insert any elevator under the retinaculum since this may scar the median nerve.
- Median nerve is now visible (Fig. 21.7a).
- Divide flexor retinaculum along its entire length under direct vision, taking care to extend beyond both pre-marked limits of the carpal tunnel (Fig. 21.7b).
- Ensure a full division has occurred distally (Fig. 21.8a) and proximally (Fig. 21.8b).

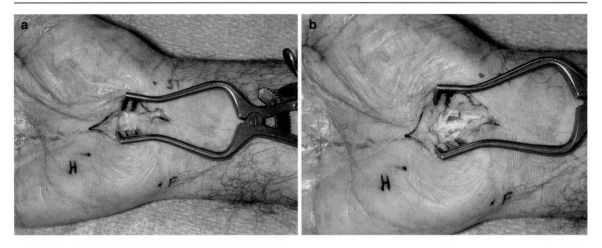

Fig. 21.6 (a) Retractor to hold skin edges apart. (b) Superficial fascia divided along line of skin incision

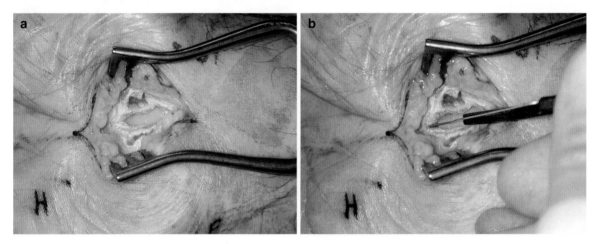

Fig. 21.7 (a) Median nerve visible under divided flexor retinaculum. (b) Ensure flexor retinaculum released along its entire length

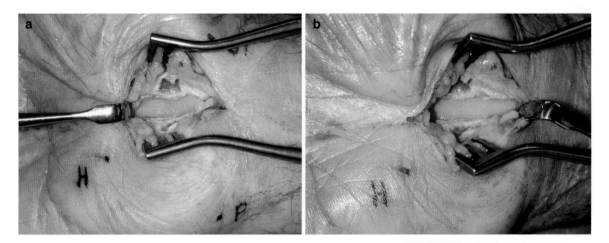

Fig. 21.8 (a) Complete the release distally. (b) Complete the release proximally

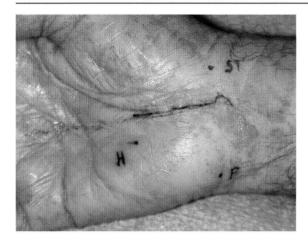

Fig. 21.9   Careful skin closure with interrupted sutures

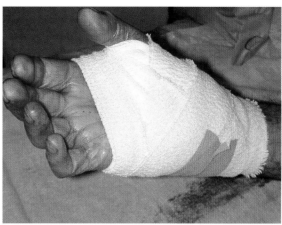

Fig. 21.10   Application of bulky bandage

Closure

- Close the skin with interrupted sutures (Fig. 21.9). Great care must be taken to prevent overlapping the skin edges on closure since this will lead to a tender and hypertrophic scar.
- Apply a bulky, padded bandage which does not extend distal to the metacarpophalangeal joints (Fig. 21.10).

Postoperative Rehabilitation

- Reduce/remove bandage at 10–12 days.
- Remove sutures if nonabsorbable.
- Encourage regular and vigorous self-massage of scar to reduce tenderness.

Outpatient Review

- Wound check at 10–12 days (wound likely to be red, even if healthy).

- Document sensory and motor function/recovery.
- Document changes in nocturnal symptoms.
- All reviews can be undertaken by GP.

Further Reading

Keith MW, Masear V, Amadio PC, et al. Treatment of carpal tunnel syndrome. J Am Acad Orthop Surg. 2009;17(6): 397–405.

Scholten RJ, Mink van der Molen A, Uitdehaag BM, et al. Surgical treatment options for carpal tunnel syndrome. Cochrane Database Syst Rev. 2007;(4):CD003905.

Benson LS, Bare AA, Nagle DJ, et al. Complications of endoscopic and open carpal tunnel release. Arthroscopy. 2006;22(9):919–24.

Uchiyama S, Itsubo T, Nakamura K, et al. Current concepts of carpal tunnel syndrome: pathophysiology, treatment, and evaluation. J Orthop Sci. 2010;15(1):1–13.

Release of the First Extensor Compartment at the Wrist (DeQuervain's Decompression)

22

Robert Farnell

Indications

- DeQuervain's disease that has not responded to nonoperative treatment including:
  - Activity modification
  - Splinting
  - Physiotherapy
  - Steroid injection

Contraindications

- Active infection
- CRPS

Preoperative Planning

Clinical Assessment

- Ensure the DeQuervain's disease remains symptomatic and Finklestein's test is positive.

Radiological Assessment

- X-rays are not necessary unless the diagnosis is in doubt.

R. Farnell
Department of Trauma and Orthopaedic Surgery,
Leeds Teaching Hospitals NHS Trust,
Leeds, UK
e-mail: robert.farnell@leedsth.nhs.uk

Preoperative Consent

- Fully explain the procedure and that there will be a permanent visible scar.
- Discuss the postoperative risks including wound infection, wrist stiffness, bleeding, and injury to the radial sensory nerve (usually temporary numbness or paresthesia but it can be permanent with hypersensitivity).
- Mark the limb.

Operative Treatment

Anesthesia

- Local anesthetic infiltration into the operative area. Bupivacaine 0.5% with adrenaline will provide a long-acting anesthetic block and reduce the risk of postoperative bleeding.

Equipment

- Standard hand surgical equipment tray
- Bipolar diathermy

Patient Positioning

- Patient supine with the arm lying on an arm table attached to the operating table.
- Fit a high arm pneumatic tourniquet.

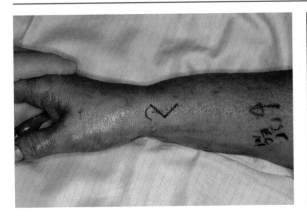

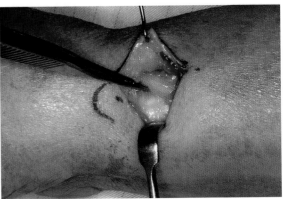

Fig. 22.1 Skin marking showing the radial styloid, direction of first extensor compartment tendons (*dotted line*), and chevron skin incision site

Fig. 22.2 Skin incision with dissection of subcutaneous fat. A large sensory branch of the radial nerve seen dorsal to the forceps

Draping and Surgical Approach

- Prepare the skin of the hand, forearm, and upper arm to the level of the tourniquet using your usual antiseptic solutions (e.g., aqueous povidone-iodine).
- Use an upper extremity exclusion drape which also covers the arm table.
- Identify the radial styloid and palpate the direction of the first extensor tendons (abductor pollicis longus (APL) and extensor pollicis brevis (EPB) tendons). Draw your skin incision with a skin marking pen. The incision can be longitudinal, transverse, or a chevron incision as used in this case (Fig. 22.1).
- Use toothed forceps to check that the operative area is anesthetized. Top up with local anesthetic if necessary.
- Exsanguinate the arm using a sterile Esmarch bandage – this is done at the last possible minute to minimize the time that the tourniquet is inflated and reduce discomfort.
- Use blunt dissection with scissors to divide the subcutaneous fat down to the extensor retinaculum. Identify and gently retract/protect branches of the sensory radial nerve and cephalic vein (Fig. 22.2).
- Use bipolar diathermy to cauterize visible vessels.

Procedure

- You will see the first extensor tendon compartment containing the APL and EPB tendons. This compartment runs from the radial styloid proximally for approximately 2 cm (Fig. 22.3a).

- Divide the extensor retinaculum which forms the roof of the first extensor compartment (Fig. 22.3b, c).
- Ensure that the APL and EPB tendons are both in the same compartment as they may lie in separate compartments (Fig. 22.4a). The APL may be made of several separate tendons which can mislead the surgeon into thinking this is also the EPB tendon. Look at the distal ends of these tendons as they leave their compartments by the radial styloid. The number of tendons can be easily seen, and you can ensure that they are not in different compartments. If they are seen to be in separate compartments, ensure that both are released (Fig. 22.4b, c).

Closure

- Skin is closed, in this case, with a single subcuticular 3/0 Prolene suture (Fig. 22.5).
- Dress with petroleum jelly gauze, dressing gauze, Velband, and a crepe bandage. Ensure the bandage only extends distally to the level of the metacarpophalangeal joints so the fingers can move freely (Fig. 22.6).
- Release the tourniquet.

Postoperative Rehabilitation

- Encourage immediate finger mobilization and elevate in a sling for 48 h.
- Simple analgesia with paracetamol if required.
- Suture and dressing removal at 2 weeks.
- Advice on scar massage with moisturizer.

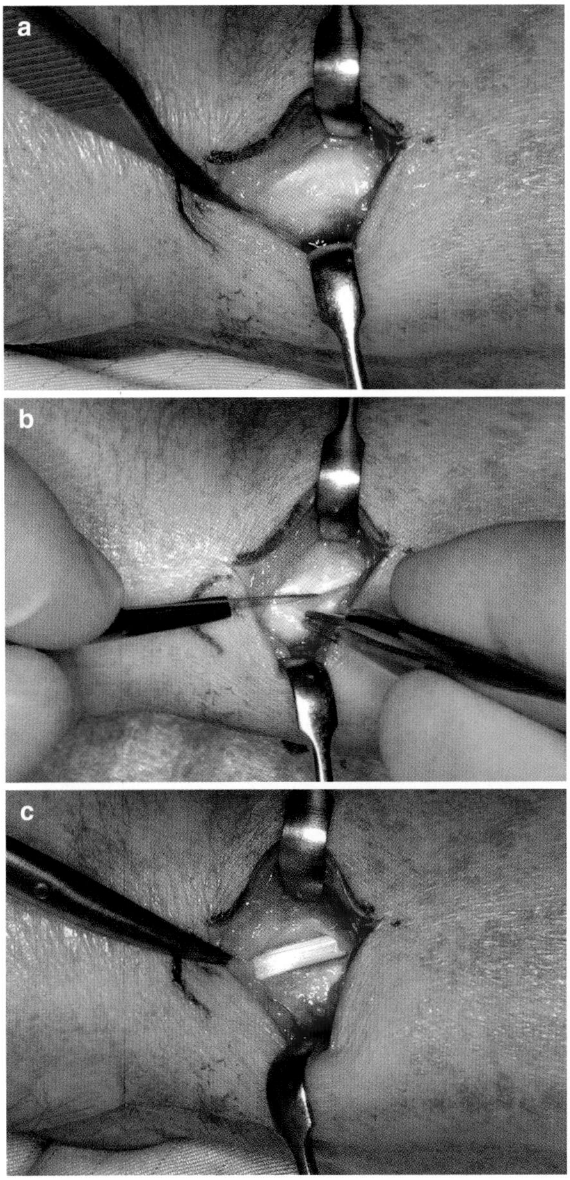

Fig. 22.3 (a) The first extensor compartment is seen after gentle retraction of the radial sensory nerve. The extensor tendons can be seen lying beneath. (b) The roof of the first extensor compartment is divided with a blade along the line of the compartment. (c) First extensor tendon compartment has been opened, but in this case, there is only one tendon lying in it. This is the EPB tendon

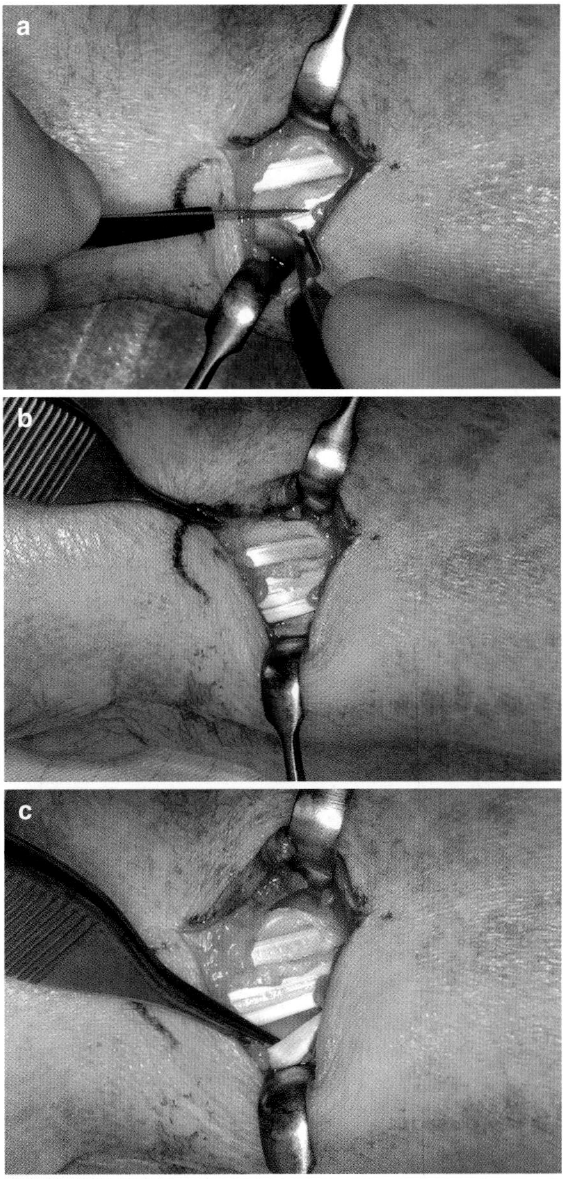

Fig. 22.4 (a) A separate compartment for the APL tendon is found beside the already opened EPB compartment, and this is opened. (b) The separate APL and EPB compartments can be seen, and (c) note that in this patient there are multiple APL tendons. If this compartment had been opened first, the surgeon may have been fooled into thinking that these were the APL and EPB tendons and ended the operation. We know the EPB tendon was in a separate compartment, and had it not been released, there is a risk that the patient's symptoms would have persisted

Outpatient Follow-up

- 2 weeks:
  - Suture removal (this can be done by the practice nurse)

- 6–8 weeks:
  - Ensure symptoms are improving.
  - Routine follow-up after this not usually required.

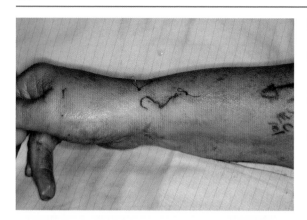

Fig. 22.5 Skin closure using a subcuticular 3/0 Prolene suture

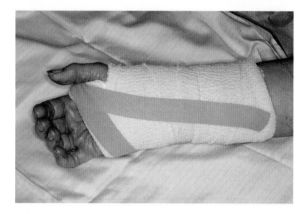

Fig. 22.6 Bandage applied. Note how this does not extend beyond the level of the MCP joints so that free finger movement is permitted

Further Reading

Scheller A, Schuh R, Hönle W, et al. Long-term results of surgical release of de Quervain's stenosing tenosynovitis. Int Orthop. 2009;33(5):1301–3.

Bouras Y, El Andaloussi Y, Zaouari T, et al. Surgical treatment in De Quervain's tenosynovitis. About 20 cases. Ann Chir Plast Esthet. 2010;55(1):42–5.

Stanley J. Radial tunnel syndrome: a surgeon's perspective. J Hand Ther. 2006;19(2):180–4.

Dupuytren's Fasciectomy

23

Doug A. Campbell

Indications

- Symptomatic functional disturbance from a Dupuytren's contracture.

Preoperative Planning

Clinical Assessment

- Decision about treatment based entirely on patient's level of functional disturbance.
- Involvement of interphalangeal joints makes surgical release more demanding.
- Assess preoperative sensation in radial and ulnar pulps of affected digits.
- Assess radial and ulnar digital artery flow by a digital Allen's test.
- Assess involvement of overlying skin in underlying contracture (Fig. 23.1a, b).
- Make decision about need for skin grafting based on level of skin involvement, recurrent, or aggressive disease.
- Discuss possible complications of:
  - Incomplete correction
  - Recurrence (inevitable in time)
  - Nerve injury (1% permanent)
  - Vascular injury
  - Infection
  - Stiffness
  - Wound breakdown

Operative Procedure

Incision

- A straight incision (seen in the ring finger) is permissible only if subsequent Z-plasty is planned (Fig. 23.2).
- A Brunner incision (seen in the little finger) – zigzag between digital flexion creases – is the standard incision for many.

Anesthesia

- Regional or general anesthetic is necessary.

Equipment

- A standard set of fine surgical instruments including scissors, fine-toothed forceps, self-retaining retractor, handheld small retractor, needle holders.
- Skin hooks and a hand table are necessary to retract skin flaps atraumatically.

Patient Positioning

- Supine.
- Affected arm on hand table.
- Ensure patient comfort before inflating tourniquet.

D.A. Campbell
Department of Trauma and Orthopaedic Surgery,
Leeds Teaching Hospitals NHS Trust,
Leeds, UK
e-mail: doug.campbell@leedsth.nhs.uk

P.V. Giannoudis (ed.), *Practical Procedures in Elective Orthopaedic Surgery*,
DOI 10.1007/978-0-85729-820-1_23, © Springer-Verlag London Limited 2012

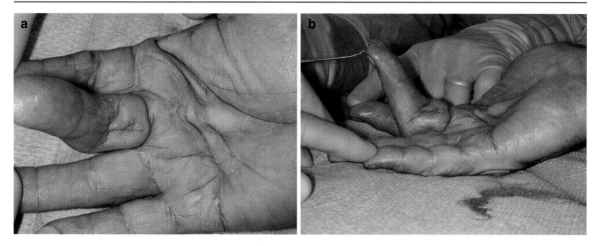

Fig. 23.1 (**a**) Dupuytren's contracture affecting overlying skin. (**b**) The preoperative contracture is seen to be 60° at the PIP joint

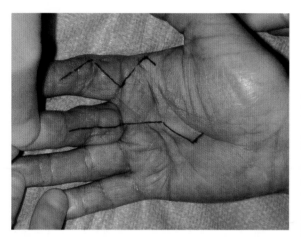

Fig. 23.2 Straight incision (*middle finger*) requires subsequent Z-plasty. Brunner incision (*index finger*) does not

Draping and Surgical Approach

- Above elbow tourniquet cuff.
- Sterile drape wrapped around upper arm at level of tourniquet cuff.
- Arm exsanguinated to level of tourniquet cuff.

Surgical Procedure

- The preoperative contracture is seen to be 60° at the proximal interphalangeal joint (Fig. 23.1b).
- The skin must be incised perpendicular to the skin surface to ensure correct skin flap thickness (Fig. 23.3a).

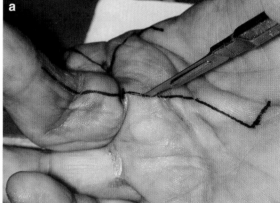

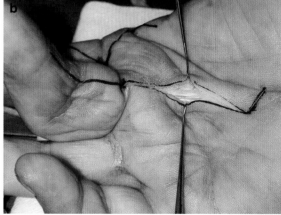

Fig. 23.3 (**a**) Perpendicular skin incisions are always made. (**b**) Careful handling of the skin edges with skin hooks

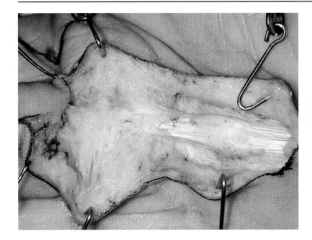

Fig. 23.4 Careful sharp dissection from the overlying skin reveals the pretendinous cord

- The skin edges are handled carefully with skin hooks (Fig. 23.3b).
- The pretendinous cord is dissected from the overlying skin by careful sharp dissection with a scalpel (Fig. 23.4).
- In the palm, the pretendinous cord lies superficial to the palmar fascia, thereby protecting the underlying neurovascular bundles from inadvertent injury.
- The cord is then divided proximally, which will partly straighten the digit (Fig. 23.5a).
- The cord is separated from the underlying superficial fascia (Fig. 23.5b, c).
- The neurovascular bundles are located on either side of the flexor tendon before they enter the digit (Fig. 23.6a).
- The neurovascular bundles are carefully and methodically traced distally into the digit, opening further skin flaps as dissection progresses (Fig. 23.6b).
- The procedure should be considered an anatomical dissection of the neurovascular bundles. In this way, these important structures will be preserved as the abnormal tissue is separated and removed.
- The scissors must be used gently. The distance between the scissor hinge and its handles is three times the distance between the hinge and the scissor tips (Fig. 23.7). Consequently, any force applied at the handles will be multiplied by three at the tips. Brutal and forceful separation of the scissor handles creates a massive and unpredictable force at the tips, creating a significant zone of injury and scarring.
- Once the correction is complete (Fig. 23.8), the Z-plasties must be created at the level of the digital

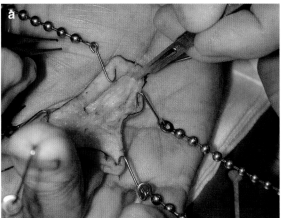
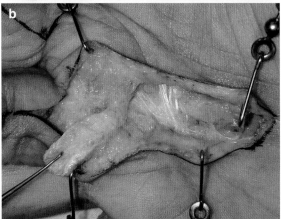
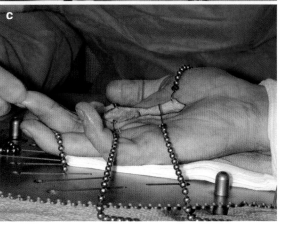

Fig. 23.5 (a) Pretendinous cord seen superficial to palmar fascia. (b) Sharp dissection releases the pretendinous cord from the superficial fascia. (c) Release of the pretendinous cord partly corrects the contracture

flexion creases. Skin marks are made at the midaxial lines at these points, and a line drawn at 60° towards the incision is made (Fig. 23.9a). These lines will form the Z-plasty incisions.

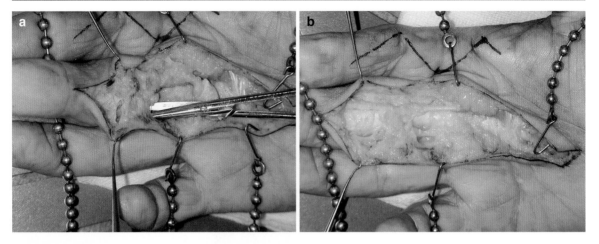

Fig. 23.6 (**a**) Both neurovascular bundles are identified adjacent to the flexor tendon. (**b**) The neurovascular bundles are carefully traced distally into the digit

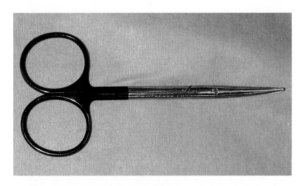

Fig. 23.7 The dissecting scissors

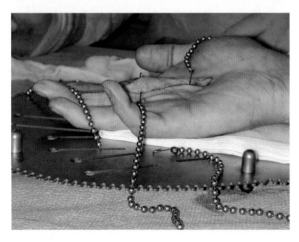

Fig. 23.8 Correction of the contracture

- Once all Z-plasty incisions have been carefully completed, the skin flaps are rearranged so that the longitudinal scar is broken up (Fig. 23.9b).

Closure

- Close the skin with interrupted sutures (Fig. 23.10). Great care must be taken to prevent overlapping the skin edges on closure since this will lead to a tender and hypertrophic scar.
- The final correction can be seen (Fig. 23.11).
- Apply a bulky, padded bandage which covers the wounds (Fig. 23.12a).
- Check the vascularity and capillary refill of the finger pulps after tourniquet release (Fig. 23.12b).

Postoperative Rehabilitation

- Reduce/remove bandage at 10–12 days.
- Remove sutures if nonabsorbable.
- Encourage regular and vigorous self-massage of scar to reduce tenderness.
- Begin early active and passive joint movements to prevent stiffness.

Outpatient Review

- Wound-check at 10–12 days (wound likely to be red, even if healthy).
- Document sensory function in radial and ulnar sides of pulp.
- Document joint positions and both active and passive ranges of motion.

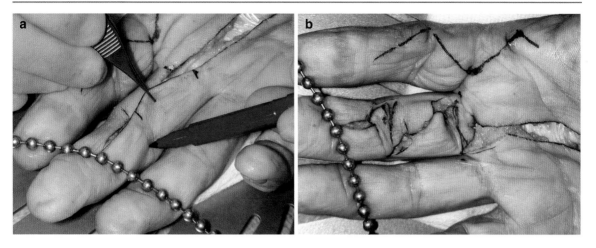

Fig. 23.9 (a) Planning lines for the Z-plasties. (b) Rearrangement of the Z-plasty skin flaps

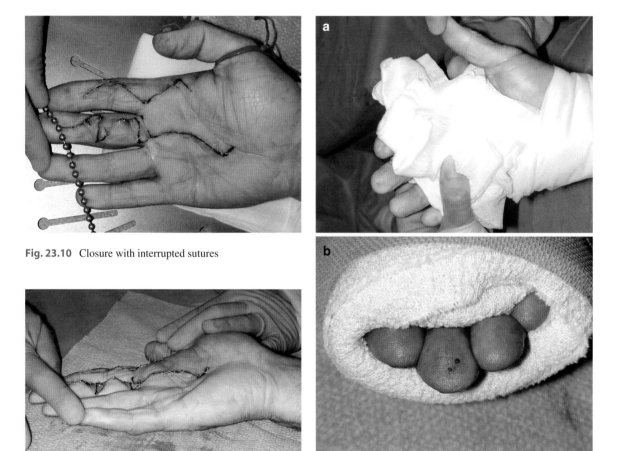

Fig. 23.10 Closure with interrupted sutures

Fig. 23.12 (a) Bulky bandage applied (b) Circulation is checked in fingertips

Fig. 23.11 Full correction of the contracture

- Refer for physiotherapy and/or night extension splints if indicated.
- Discharge when movement recovered and function restored.

Further Reading

Shaw Jr RB, Chong AK, Zhang A, et al. Dupuytren's disease: history, diagnosis, and treatment. Plast Reconstr Surg. 2007;120(3):44e–54.

Zyluk A, Jagielski W. The effect of the severity of the Dupuytren's contracture on the function of the hand before and after surgery. J Hand Surg Eur Vol. 2007;32(3):326–9.

Bulstrode NW, Jemec B, Smith PJ. The complications of Dupuytren's contracture surgery. J Hand Surg Am. 2005;30(5):1021–5.

Denkler K. Surgical complications associated with fasciectomy for Dupuytren's disease: a 20-year review of the English literature. Eplasty. 2010;10:15.

Trigger Finger Release

24

Robert Farnell

Indications

- Trigger finger/thumb that has failed to respond to nonoperative treatment.

Contraindications

- Active infection.
- CRPS.

Preoperative Planning

Clinical Assessment

- Ensure the trigger finger remains symptomatic and triggering.

Radiological Assessment

- X-rays are not necessary.

Preoperative Consent

- Fully explain the procedure and that there will be a permanent visible scar.

R. Farnell
Department of Trauma and Orthopaedic Surgery,
Leeds Teaching Hospitals NHS Trust,
Leeds, UK
e-mail: robert.farnell@leedsth.nhs.uk

- Discuss the postoperative risks including wound infection, stiffness, and injury to the digital nerves.
- Mark the finger.

Operative Treatment

Anesthesia

- Infiltration of local anesthesia (bupivacaine 0.5% or lidocaine 1%) in the palm around the planned incision.

Equipment

- Standard hand surgical equipment tray.
- Bipolar diathermy.
- Loupe magnification if you are familiar with this.

Patient Positioning

- Patient supine with the arm lying on an arm table attached to the operating table.
- Fit an upper arm pneumatic tourniquet.

Draping and Surgical Approach

- Prepare the skin of the hand, forearm, and upper arm to the level of the tourniquet using your usual antiseptic solution (e.g., aqueous povidone-iodine).
- Use an upper extremity exclusion drape which also covers the arm table (Fig. 24.1).

P.V. Giannoudis (ed.), *Practical Procedures in Elective Orthopaedic Surgery*,
DOI 10.1007/978-0-85729-820-1_24, © Springer-Verlag London Limited 2012

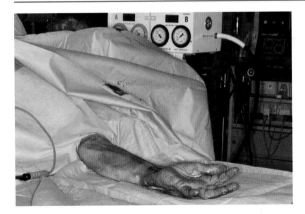

Fig. 24.1 Preparation of the arm with a pneumatic tourniquet, an arm table, and upper extremity drape

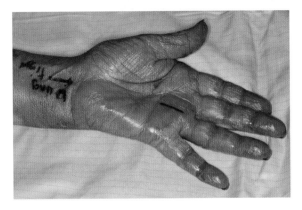

Fig. 24.2 Skin marking showing the planned skin incision site – a longitudinal incision in this case

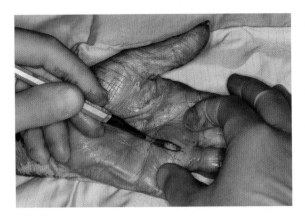

Fig. 24.3 Skin incision

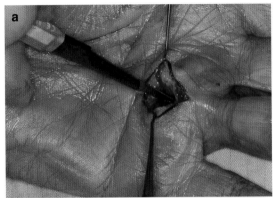

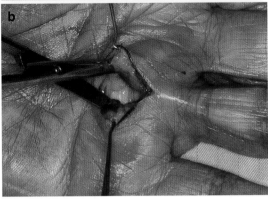

Fig. 24.4 (a) Deeper dissection using skin hooks to put the soft tissues under tension and pushing a scalpel blade into the wound. Ensure you remain in the midline. (b) Scissors can be used to complete the dissection of soft tissues off the A1 pulley

- Draw your skin incision with a skin marking pen. A longitudinal or transverse incision may be used (Fig. 24.2).
- Exsanguinate the arm using an Esmarch bandage – do this when all of the above have been done to reduce the time the tourniquet is inflated as this is uncomfortable.
- Make the skin incision and use bipolar diathermy to cauterize visible vessels (Fig. 24.3).
- Put skin hooks in the skin edges either side of the incision. Put the soft tissues under tension by pulling the edges apart and use a scalpel by pushing into the wound to divide the tissues. If you use this technique and keep the incision in the midline of the finger, you are unlikely to cause injury to nearby structures (Fig. 24.4a). At the deep extent of the

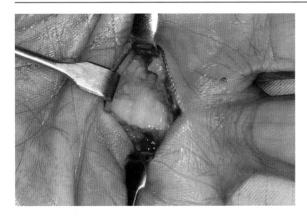

Fig. 24.5 Insert retractors to allow a clear view of the A1 pulley

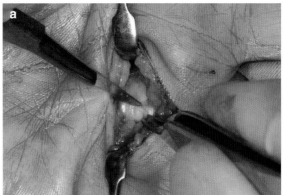

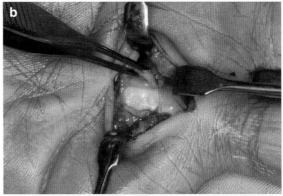

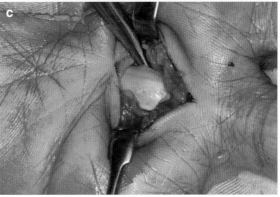

incision, use blunt dissection with scissors to clearly identify the A1 pulley in the midline (Fig. 24.4b).

Procedure

- Retract the soft tissues so that a clear view of the A1 pulley is obtained. It is not necessary to identify the neurovascular bundles so long as you have remained in the midline and you have seen all structures divided with the knife (Fig. 24.5).
- Release the A1 pulley in the midline (Fig. 24.6a). Be careful not to continue this incision too far distally and divide the A2 pulley (this is easier to do than you think especially with a longitudinal incision).
- Ensure the A1 pulley has been completely divided (Fig. 24.6b). There may be visible synovial hypertrophy around the flexor tendons (Fig. 24.6c).
- Ensure there is no further triggering by asking the patient to open and close their fingers.

Fig. 24.6 (**a**) Dividing the A1 pulley under direct vision in the midline. (**b**) The A1 pulley has been divided and is seen held in the forceps. (**c**) There is visible synovial hypertrophy around the flexor tendons

Closure

- Skin has been closed in this case using 5/0 interrupted Vicryl Rapide sutures (monofilament sutures can also be used) (Fig. 24.7).
- Dress with a non-adherent dressing such as petroleum jelly–covered gauze, dressing gauze, Velband, and a crepe bandage (Fig. 24.8a, b, c).
- Release the tourniquet and elevate in a Bradford sling.

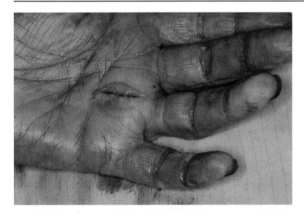

Fig. 24.7 Skin closure with interrupted 5/0 Vicryl Rapide sutures

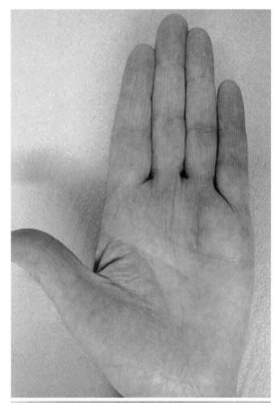

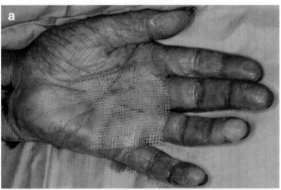

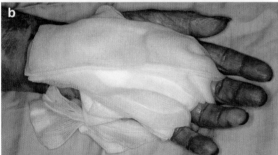

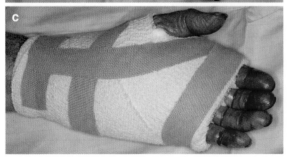

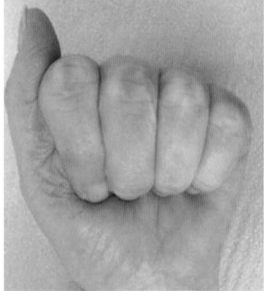

Fig. 24.9 Six weeks post surgery. The scar is difficult to see and it will fade over the next few months

Fig. 24.8 (**a**) Non-adherent dressing using petroleum jelly–covered gauze. (**b**) Dressing gauze between the fingers. (**c**) Dressing completed using Velband and a crepe bandage

Postoperative Rehabilitation

- Encourage immediate finger mobilization and elevate in a sling for 48 h.
- Simple analgesia with paracetamol if required.

Outpatient Follow-up

- 2 weeks:
  - Suture and dressing removal.
- 6 weeks:
  - Ensure symptoms are improving.
  - Advice on scar massage with moisturizer (Fig. 24.9).
  - Routine follow-up after this not usually required.

Further Reading

Makkouk AH, Oetgen ME, Swigart CR, et al. Trigger finger: etiology, evaluation, and treatment. Curr Rev Musculoskelet Med. 2008;1(2):92–6.

Ryzewicz M, Wolf JM. Trigger digits: principles, management, and complications. J Hand Surg Am. 2006;31(1):135–46.

Lange-Riess D, Schuh R, Hönle W, et al. Long-term results of surgical release of trigger finger and trigger thumb in adults. Arch Orthop Trauma Surg. 2009;129(12):1617–9.

Dierks U, Hoffmann R, Meek MF. Open versus percutaneous release of the A1-pulley for stenosing tendovaginitis: a prospective randomized trial. Tech Hand Up Extrem Surg. 2008;12(3):183–7.

Tendon Transfers for Median Nerve Palsy

25

Gráinne Bourke and Andrew Williams

Introduction

- Median nerve palsy results in loss of thumb flexion and opposition. It also results in loss of isolated flexion of the proximal interphalangeal joints of all the fingers and loss of flexion of the distal interphalangeal joints of the index and middle fingers. Sensation is lost on the palm of the hand and on the volar surface of the 3 and ½ radial digits.
- Deficits in sensation may impact significantly upon the result of restoring motor function.
- The only muscles in the flexor compartment which function following a high-level lesion are the flexor carpi ulnaris and flexor digitorum profundus to the little and ring fingers.
- In procedures designed to reproduce thumb opposition, it may be necessary to change the line of pull of the transferred tendon to restore function. Pulleys should be strong, located in the region of the pisiform, and should not cause an acute change in angle.
- The tendons affected in median nerve palsy:
  - Low lesion:
    Abductor pollicis brevis
    Opponens pollicis and the superficial head flexor pollicis brevis
    Lumbricales to index and middle fingers
  - High lesion (as above plus):
    Flexor pollicis longus
    Flexor digitorum superficialis

Flexor digitorum profundus (index and ½ middle)
Pronator quadratus
Pronator teres
Flexor carpi radialis

Indications

- Tendon transfers are used to provide active controlled motion when there is loss of motor function in the median nerve and/or the anterior interosseus nerve distribution.
- The aim of tendon transfers in median nerve palsy is to restore key pinch, which involves thumb opposition and flexion and index finger flexion.

Timing of Tendon Transfer

- At the time of nerve repair or when nerve recovery is expected to act as an internal splint.
- After failure of spontaneous nerve recovery or failure of recovery following nerve repair.
- As a substitute for nerve repair in those patients who are not suitable.

Preoperative

Clinical Assessment

- Signs of median nerve palsy
  - Absent thumb opposition and abduction
  - Absent flexion of the DIP and PIP joints of the middle and index fingers

G. Bourke (✉) • A. Williams
Department of Plastic and Reconstructive Surgery,
Leeds Teaching Hospitals NHS Trust,
Leeds, UK
e-mail: grainnebourke@nhs.net

P.V. Giannoudis (ed.), *Practical Procedures in Elective Orthopaedic Surgery*,
DOI 10.1007/978-0-85729-820-1_25, © Springer-Verlag London Limited 2012

- Absent flexion of the thumb
- Absent forearm pronation
- Weakness and ulnar deviation on wrist flexion
- A tight first web space
- Numbness of the palm and palmer surface of the radial 3 and 1/2 digits
- Essential requirements to ensure a good functional result
  - Adequate soft tissues cover to enable tendon gliding
  - A stable underlying skeleton
  - Normal or near-normal joint mobility of the wrist, fingers, and thumb
  - The musculotendinous units to be used for transfer are expendable and have adequate power and excursion
  - A cooperative and reliable patient
- Notes
  - Intrinsic recovery is less predictable and less likely than extrinsic recovery
  - Thumb opposition and abduction may be preserved by an anomalous nerve supply from the ulnar nerve
  - The loss of sensation significantly influences the motor recovery with regard to grip strength and function
  - The patient will rely on visual input to supplement sensory recovery when using the hand
- Opposition transfers
  - *Royle-Thompson* – flexor digitorum superficialis 4 through palmar fascia sling to abductor pollicis brevis or extensor pollicis brevis
  - *Bunnell* – FDS 4 through flexor carpi ulnaris sling to abductor pollicis brevis or extensor pollicis brevis
  - *Burkhalter* – extensor indicis around ulnar wrist to abductor pollicis brevis or extensor pollicis brevis
  - *Camitz* transfer – palmaris longus with palmar fascia to abductor pollicis brevis
  - *Huber* transfer – abductor digiti minimi to abductor pollicis brevis or extensor pollicis brevis
  - Extensor digiti minimi around ulnar border wrist to abductor pollicis brevis, extensor expansion, and extensor pollicis longus
- Transfers for thumb flexion
  - Brachioradialis to flexor pollicis longus
  - Extensor carpi radialis longus/extensor carpi radialis brevis to flexor pollicis longus

- Transfers for index and middle finger flexion
  - Intact ulnar flexor digitorum profundus side-to-side
  - Extensor carpi radialis longus to flexor digitorum profundus
- Transfers for Forearm Pronation
  - Zancolli rerouting of the biceps tendon

Operative Procedure

- All procedures are performed under general anesthesia.
- The patient is placed in a supine position with the arm extended on a hand table.
- A pneumatic tourniquet is applied to the upper arm. The cuff is inflated to 100 mmHg above systolic blood pressure.
- Specialist equipment:
  - A tendon braider to enable Pulvertaft weave.
  - A Carroll tendon retriever to enable smooth passage of tendons.
  - All tendon repairs are performed with 3–0 nonabsorbable sutures.

Opponensplasties

Flexor Digitorum Superficialis

- A transverse incision is made at the base of either the ring or the middle finger on the volar surface. The flexor digitorum superficialis tendon is located through a window between the A1 and A2 pulleys (Fig. 25.1a).
- With the finger flexed, the flexor digitorum superficialis is divided proximal to Camper's chiasm. This remaining distal 1 cm of flexor digitorum superficialis prevents the development of a swan-neck deformity (Fig. 25.1b).

Royle-Thompson

- An incision is made along the radial border of the hypothenar eminence, through which the ulnar edge of the palmar aponeurosis is identified (Fig. 25.2).
- The divided flexor digitorum superficialis tendon is brought out through this palmar incision.
- Another incision is made over the dorsum of the thumb metacarpophalangeal joint. A subcutaneous

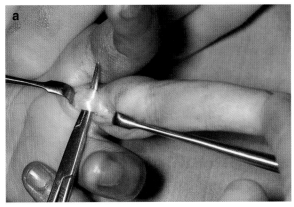

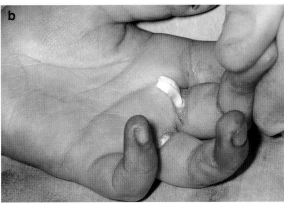

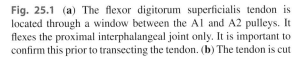

Fig. 25.1 (**a**) The flexor digitorum superficialis tendon is located through a window between the A1 and A2 pulleys. It flexes the proximal interphalangeal joint only. It is important to confirm this prior to transecting the tendon. (**b**) The tendon is cut proximal to Camper's chiasm. The remaining distal 1 cm of flexor digitorum superficialis, as illustrated here, prevents the development of a swan-neck deformity

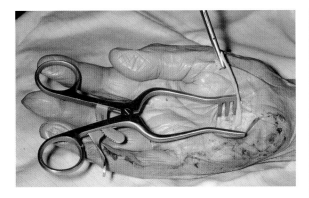

Fig. 25.2 An incision is made along the radial border of the hypothenar eminence, through which the ulnar edge of the palmar aponeurosis is identified. This acts as a pulley for the divided flexor digitorum superficialis tendon which is retrieved through this incision prior to being redirected toward the thumb

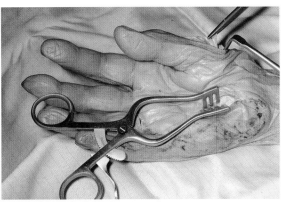

Fig. 25.3 A subcutaneous tunnel is formed between the palmar incision and the thumb. The tendon is passed through this tunnel and then sutured to the insertion of the abductor pollicis brevis

tunnel is dissected between this and the palmar incision.
- The flexor digitorum superficialis is passed through the tunnel, with the ulnar border of the palmar aponeurosis and the distal flexor retinaculum acting as the pulley (Fig. 25.3).
- Alternatively, an incision is made in the distal forearm, proximal to the pisiform. The flexor carpi ulnaris is identified. A distally based loop of flexor carpi ulnaris is created from 20% of the tendon by suturing it to itself. The flexor digitorum superficialis is brought out of the carpal tunnel passed through the loop and then through the subcutaneous tunnel to the thumb metacarpophalangeal joint.

- The flexor digitorum superficialis tendon is attached under full tension to the abductor pollicis brevis with the wrist in neutral and the thumb held in opposition.
- The wounds are closed and dressed.

Bunnell's

- An incision is made proximal to the wrist crease over the ulnar neurovascular bundle exposing the distal flexor carpi ulnaris.
- The flexor carpi ulnaris is split longitudinally proximal to its insertion and then looped back on itself to

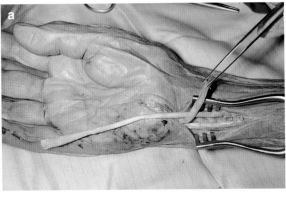
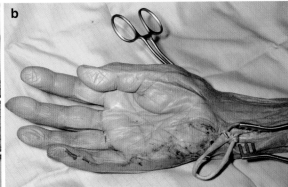

Fig. 25.4 (**a**) The flexor tendon is retrieved in the wrist through an ulnar incision. A strip of flexor carpi ulnaris is cut proximally and sutured to itself to form a pulley. This enables the redirection of the transferred tendon toward the thumb. (**b**) The flexor digitorum brevis tendon is then passed subcutaneously toward the thumb and sutured to the insertion of the abductor pollicis brevis

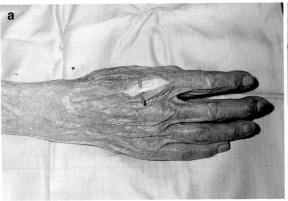
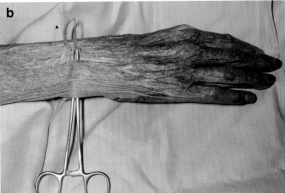

Fig. 25.5 (**a**) The extensor indicis is harvested at the level of the index metacarpophalangeal joint. This is located ulnar to the tendon of extensor digitorum communis. (**b**) The extensor indi-cis is then retrieved through a longitudinal incision proximal to the extensor retinaculum before being transferred around the ulnar border of the wrist

create a pulley for the flexor digitorum superficialis (Fig. 25.4a).
- An incision is made over the dorsum of the thumb metacarpophalangeal joint and a subcutaneous tunnel dissected between this and the wrist incision.
- The divided flexor digitorum superficialis tendon is delivered into the wrist incision, passed through the pulley in flexor carpi ulnaris, and then through the subcutaneous tunnel to the thumb (Fig. 25.4b).
- A hole is drilled in the proximal phalanx of the thumb from the dorsoulnar to the radial cortex. This must be large enough for the transferred tendon to pass through.
- The flexor digitorum superficialis is passed dorsally over of extensor pollicis longus and through the hole in the proximal phalanx.

- The tension is adjusted so that the thumb lies in full opposition with the wrist in neutral, and the flexor digitorum superficialis is sutured to itself or to the radial periosteum.
- The wounds are closed and dressed.

Notes

- The middle finger flexor digitorum superficialis may be preferred as a donor over the ring finger so as not to weaken grip strength.
- The ring finger flexor digitorum superficialis may not be available in high median nerve injuries.
- The ring finger flexor digitorum superficialis should not be used in individuals with combined low

median and high ulnar nerve injuries as this is the only ring finger flexor.

- The ring finger flexor digitorum superficialis may also be required for the treatment of claw deformity in ulnar nerve lesions.

Extensor Indicis Opponensplasty

- A longitudinal incision is made over the index finger metacarpophalangeal joint, and the extensor indicis, lying ulnar to the extensor communis tendon, is divided just proximal to the extensor hood (Fig. 25.5a).
- Another incision is made on the dorsoulnar aspect of the distal forearm.
- The extensor indicis is delivered from underneath the extensor retinaculum where it can be freed from its adhesions (Fig. 25.5b).
- A further incision is made over the radial border of the thumb metacarpophalangeal joint.
- A subcutaneous tunnel is developed across the palm and around the ulnar border of the wrist and forearm to the dorsoulnar forearm incision.
- The extensor indicis is passed through this tunnel, superficial to extensor carpi ulnaris and flexor carpi ulnaris.
- The transfer is sutured to the abductor pollicis brevis under maximal tension with the wrist in 30° of flexion and the thumb in full opposition.
- The wounds are closed and dressed.

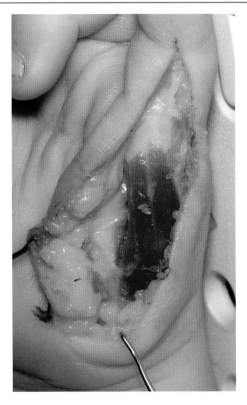

Fig. 25.6 The abductor digiti minimi is raised through an incision along the ulnar border of the little finger and hypothenar eminence. Proximally, the incision curves radially over the hypothenar muscles. It is important to harvest the full length of the tendon to have enough length for subsequent transfer

Notes

- This transfer has the advantage of not weakening grip.
- It can be used when the flexor digitorum superficialis muscle unit is not available.
- Its loss does not impair hand function.
- It can be used in combined median and ulnar nerve injuries.

Abductor Digiti Minimi Opponensplasty (Huber)

- A long curvilinear incision is made from the PIPJ of the ulnar border of the little finger, across the radial border of the hypothenar eminence (Fig. 25.6).

- The abductor digiti minimi is divided from its insertion and dissected in a retrograde fashion toward its origin from the pisiform.
- Care must be taken proximally where its pedicle enters on the radial surface.
- The origin may be preserved, but if extra length is required, it can be divided leaving only an attachment to the flexor carpi ulnaris and the neurovascular pedicle intact.
- Another incision is made over the radial border of the thumb metacarpophalangeal joint, and a subcutaneous tunnel, developed between this and the wrist incision.
- The abductor digiti minimi is passed through the tunnel and attached to the abductor pollicis brevis with the thumb in full opposition.
- The wounds are closed and dressed.

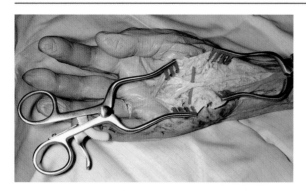

Fig. 25.7 This cadaver dissection illustrates the palmaris longus tendon which has been dissected proximal to the wrist crease and distally into the palm. This tendon can then be cut distally and transferred subcutaneously to the thumb to enable abduction

Notes

- This transfer improves the cosmesis as well as the function of the hand by adding muscle volume to the thenar eminence.

Palmaris Longus Opponensplasty (Camitz)

- A standard carpal tunnel incision is extended 2 cm proximally and the carpal tunnel decompressed.
- The palmaris longus tendon is identified and dissected in continuity with a strip of palmar aponeurosis (Fig. 25.7).
- A further incision is made over the radial border of the thumb metacarpophalangeal joint, and a subcutaneous tunnel, developed between this and the wrist incision superficial to the thenar musculature.
- The palmaris longus is passed through the tunnel and weaved to the abductor pollicis brevis under maximal tension with the thumb in full opposition, the metacarpophalangeal joint extended, and the wrist in neutral.
- The wounds are closed and dressed.

Notes

- This transfer is best performed at the time of carpal tunnel decompression for individuals who lack thumb abduction due to injury of the median nerve caused by compression at this level.

Opponensplasty Insertions

- Single insertion techniques
  - The abductor pollicis brevis insertion is used in isolated median nerve injuries.
- Dual insertion techniques
  - Opposition and stabilization of MCPJ or inhibition of IPJ flexion. The transfer will tend to act predominantly on the function which is performed under greatest tension.

Postoperative Management for Opponensplasty

- The thumb is held in opposition in a rigid cast splint for 4 weeks.
- At 4 weeks, the sutures are removed and a thermoplastic splint holding the thumb in opposition is amade.
- A therapist should then commence a reeducation program, stressing synergistic movements.

Follow-up

- At 3, 6, and 12 months will allow the success of the procedure to be assessed.

Digit Flexion Transfers in High Median Nerve Lesions

Extensor Carpi Radialis Longus to Flexor Digitorum Profundus of the Index

- A dorsoradial incision based over the wrist is made over the extensor carpi radialis longus.
- The extensor carpi radialis longus is detached from its insertion on the second metacarpal.
- The tendon is then tunneled subcutaneously around the radial border of the wrist to the midline.
- The tendon is woven into the flexor digitorum profundus of the index ± middle fingers.
- The tension should be set such that the finger is fully flexed with 30° of wrist extension and fully extended with 30° of wrist flexion.

Brachioradialis to Flexor Pollicis Longus

- A volar radial incision is used to perform this transfer.
- The insertion of the brachioradialis onto the distal radius is cut, and the brachioradialis is freed from its proximal fascial attachments in the forearm to enable better excursion.
- The adjacent flexor pollicis longus tendon is identified.
- The brachioradialis tendon is woven into the flexor pollicis longus tendon proximal to the carpal tunnel.
- The tension should be set such that with the wrist flexed at 30°, the thumb IPJ, MCPJ, and CMCJ can be passively extended.
- In this position, the IPJ will not fully flex, but this is not functionally essential.

Notes

- Careful consideration needs to be given as to whether any significant functional improvement will be achieved in high median nerve palsies by performing tendon transfers.
- If the ulnar nerve is intact, flexion of the index finger is best restored by suturing of the index flexor digitorum profundus to the conjoint middle, ring, and little flexor digitorum profundus tendons in the distal forearm.
- Tendon transfers for median nerve palsy are usually performed end-to-side so that any recovery of nerve function does not compromise normal functioning of the original motor unit.
- The excursion of the available donor units (extensor carpi radialis longus, extensor carpi ulnaris, and brachioradialis) is significantly less than the digital flexor tendons.
- To maximize finger flexion, the wrist must be extended and the wrist flexed for digit extension.
- If strength of index flexion is required, the extensor carpi radialis longus transfer can be transferred to the index flexor digitorum profundus.
- For the brachioradialis to adequately flex the thumb, it must be freed of all its attachments in the distal two-third of the forearm.
- Brachioradialis crosses the elbow joint; the thumb position will be influenced by the tenodesis effect across this joint.

Further Reading

Bunnell S. Opposition of the thumb. J Bone Joint Surg. 1938;20:269.

Cooney WP. Tendon transfer for median nerve palsy. Hand Clin. 1988;4(2):155.

Green DP, Hotchkiss RN, Pederson WC, Wolfe SW. Green's operative hand surgery. 5th ed. New York: Churchill Livingstone; 2005.

Scheker L, Cendales LC. Correcting congenital thumb anomalies in children – opponensplasty and pollicization. In: Gupta A, Kay SPJ, Scheker LR, editors. The growing hand: diagnosis and management of the upper extremity in children. London: Mosby; 2000.

Cawrse NH, Sammut D. A modification in technique of abductor digiti minimi (Huber) opponensplasty. J Hand Surg BR. 1991;16(1):56–60.

Tendon Transfers for Radial Nerve Palsy

26

Gráinne Bourke and Andrew Williams

Introduction

- Radial nerve palsy causes loss of wrist, finger, and thumb extension as well as loss of supination with the arm extended. This leads to a lack of grip strength. The sensory impairment is usually confined to the snuff box or dorsal aspect of the first web space.
- The tendons affected in radial nerve palsy:
  – Extensor carpi radialis longus
  – Extensor carpi radialis brevis
  – Brachioradialis
  – Supinator
  – Extensor digitorum communis
  – Extensor pollicis longus
  – Abductor pollicis longus
- The tendons affected in posterior interosseous nerve palsy:
  – Extensor digitorum communis
  – Extensor pollicis longus
  – Abductor pollicis longus

Indications

- Tendon transfers are used to provide active controlled motion when there is loss of motor function in the radial nerve and\or the posterior interosseous nerve distribution.

Timing of Tendon Transfer

- At the time of nerve repair or when nerve recovery is expected to act as an internal splint.
- After failure of spontaneous nerve recovery or failure of recovery following nerve repair.
- As a substitute for nerve repair in those patients who are not suitable.

Preoperative Planning

Clinical Assessment

Signs of Radial Nerve Palsy
- Lack of wrist, digit, and thumb extension.
- Weakness of grip strength.
- Altered sensation in the anatomical snuff box and first web space dorsally.

Essential Requirements to Ensure a Good Functional Result
- Adequate soft tissues cover to enable tendon gliding.
- A stable underlying skeleton.
- Normal or near normal joint mobility of the wrist, fingers, and thumb.

G. Bourke (✉) • A. Williams
Department of Plastic and Reconstructive Surgery,
Leeds Teaching Hospitals NHS Trust,
Leeds, UK
e-mail: grainnebourke@nhs.net

P.V. Giannoudis (ed.), *Practical Procedures in Elective Orthopaedic Surgery*,
DOI 10.1007/978-0-85729-820-1_26, © Springer-Verlag London Limited 2012

Fig. 26.1 (**a**) A Carroll tendon retriever. (**b**) A tendon braider to enable tendon weaving

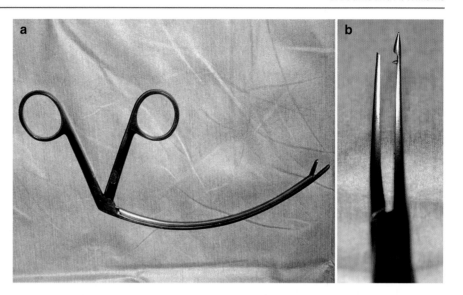

- The musculotendinous units to be used for transfer are expendable and have adequate power and excursion.
- A cooperative and reliable patient.

Tendon Transfer Options

Brand Transfers

- Pronator teres to extensor carpi radialis brevis (high level palsy).
- Flexor carpi radialis to extensor digitorum communis 2–5 (Starr)/flexor carpi ulnaris to extensor digitorum communis 2–5 (Jones).
- Palmaris longus to extensor pollicis longus.

Boyes Transfers

- Pronator teres to extensor carpi radialis longus and extensor carpi radialis brevis (high level palsy).
- Flexor digitorum superficialis 3 to extensor digitorum communis (via interosseous membrane).
- Flexor digitorum superficialis 4 to extensor indices proprius and extensor pollicis longus (via interosseous membrane).
- Flexor carpi radialis to abductor pollicis longus and extensor pollicis brevis.

Note

In Posterior Interosseous Nerve Palsy

- The unopposed action of extensor carpi longus causes radial deviation of the wrist. This may be corrected by side-to-side repair of extensor carpi radialis longus to extensor carpi radialis brevis.
- Flexor carpi ulnaris should be preserved to avoid worsening radial deviation of wrist extension.

Operative Procedure for Complete Radial Nerve Palsy Above the Elbow

- All procedures are performed under general anesthesia or brachial plexus block.
- The patient is placed in a supine position with the arm extended on a hand table.
- A pneumatic tourniquet is applied to the upper arm. The cuff is inflated to 100 mmHg above systolic blood pressure.
- Specialist equipment:
  - A Carroll tendon retriever to enable smooth passage of tendon from the volar to dorsal forearm (Fig. 26.1a).
  - A tendon braider to enable Pulvertaft weave (Fig. 26.1b).
  - All tendon repairs are performed with 3–0 nonabsorbable sutures.

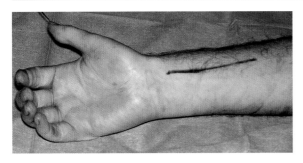

Fig. 26.2 A longitudinal incision on radial aspect of the volar forearm

Operative Procedure

Transfers for Wrist Extension, Finger Extension, and Thumb Extension

- *Pronator teres to extensor carpi radialis brevis.*
- *Flexor carpi radialis to extensor digitorum communis.*
- *Palmaris longus to extensor pollicis longus.*
  - A radial incision is made on the volar aspect of the forearm, exposing the underlying flexor tendons (Fig. 26.2).
  - The tendons of palmaris longus, flexor carpi radialis, and brachioradialis are dissected from ulnar to radial. The sensory branch of the radial nerve is preserved lying adjacent to the brachioradialis tendon(Fig. 26.3a).
  - The short tendon of pronator teres is found inserting onto the radius by radially retracting the brachioradialis tendon.
  - A periosteal strip is dissected and harvested with the pronator teres to augment the tendon length (Fig. 26.3b).
  - A dorsal incision is then made to identify the recipient tendons (Fig. 26.4). This is centered over the fourth dorsal compartment (extensor digitorum communis) and can be extended proximally and/or distally to ensure adequate access to the wrist extensors (second dorsal compartment) and the extensor pollicis longus (thirddorsal compartment).
  - The extensor carpi radialis brevis is dissected. This inserts into the third metacarpal base and is thus the most central wrist extensor.

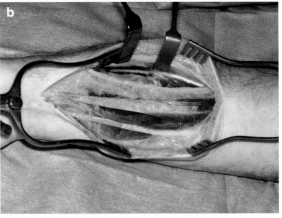

Fig. 26.3 (**a**) The tendons of palmaris longus, flexor carpi radialis, and brachioradialis. The cutaneous radial nerve is clearly seen between flexor carpi radialis and brachioradialis. (**b**) A strip of periosteum is dissected with the tendon of pronator teres

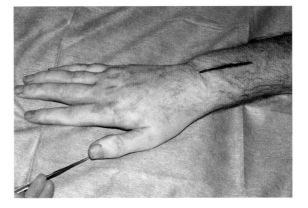

Fig. 26.4 Dorsal incision

- The tendon of pronator teres is passed, in a subcutaneous tunnel, lying superficial to the brachioradialis to the extensor carpi radialis brevis. The periosteal extension harvested with the tendon is essential to allow adequate tendon overlapping in the Pulvertaft weave to ensure a robust repair.
- The tendons may be repaired end to end (when there is full paralysis and no further recovery of the radial nerve is expected) or end to side (to act as an internal splint while waiting for nerve regeneration and recovery).
- The tendons of the extensor digitorum communis and extensor pollicis longus are dissected (Fig. 26.5).
- The extensor pollicis longus must be dissected free from its course around Lister's tubercle. It is important to dissect this tendon proximally to the musculotendinous junction.
- The tendon of flexor carpi radialis is divided distally at the wrist (Fig. 26.6).
- It is rerouted subcutaneously around the radial border of the forearm and secured o the extensor digitorum communis either end to end (when there is full paralysis of the radial nerve and no further recovery of the radial nerve is expected) or end to side (to act as an internal splint while waiting for nerve regeneration and recovery) (Fig. 26.7).
- The palmaris longus is dissected and cut distally at the wrist. The Extensor pollicis longus is cut at the musculotendinous junction and rerouted radially to join the palmaris longus. This yields an abducted position for the thumb and improves the first web space. This will improve thumb function (Fig. 26.8).
- Closure is performed in two layers with absorbable sutures (Fig. 26.9a, b). The wounds are dressed.
- A plaster of Paris splint is fashioned to maintain the forearm in 15–30° of pronation, the wrist in 45° of extension, the MCPJs in 10–15° of flexion, and the thumb in maximal extension and abduction.

Notes

- If palmaris longus is absent, then the extensor pollicis longus can be joined to the flexor carpi radialis – extensor digitorum communis transfer (Fig. 26.10).

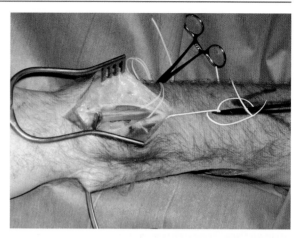

Fig. 26.5 The pale paralyzed musculotendinous junctions of the extensor digitorum communis (*yellow*) and extensor pollicis longus(*white*) are identified

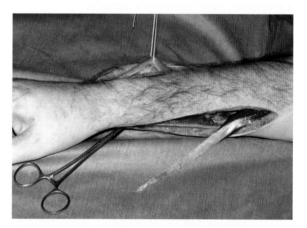

Fig. 26.6 Flexor carpi radialis is cut distally at the wrist

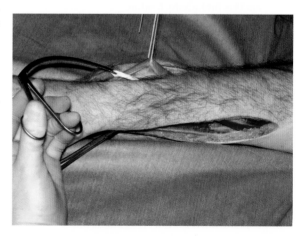

Fig. 26.7 Flexor carpi radialis is passed through a subcutaneous tunnel on the radial aspect of the forearm to power the extensor digitorum communis

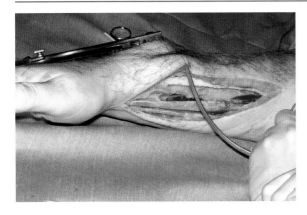

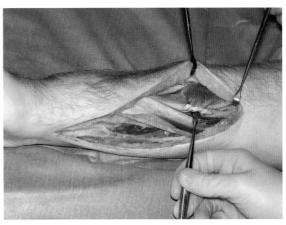

Fig. 26.8 Extensor carpi radialis brevis is passed through a subcutaneous tunnel toward the periosteal extension of pronator teres

Fig. 26.10 Pronator teres is sutured to extensor carpi radialis brevis, with the tendons of flexor carpi radialis and palmaris longus passing subcutaneously around the radial border of the forearm to the extensor digitorum communis and the extensor pollicis longus, respectively

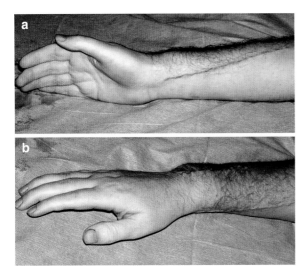

Fig. 26.9 (a, b) The wounds are closed

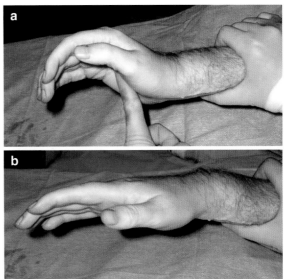

Fig. 26.11 (a) The fingers and thumb are extended with the wrist in slight flexion, (b) with the wrist extended and the fingers and thumb still flexed, indicating the transfer is not too tight

- The correct tension is achieved with the wrist and fingers in neutral and maximal tension on the flexor carpi radialis.
- Securing the transfers with adequate tension is difficult to judge, and it is essential that full extension can be achieved while not restricting flexion of the digits and wrist.
- In general, extensor tendon transfers will stretch slightly with time and should therefore be secured tightly.
- Upon completion, with the wrist flexed, the fingers and thumb should fully extend but not hyperextend, and with the wrist extended, it should still be possible to flex the fingers into the palm.

- If the line of pull of the FCR is not satisfactory, it can be brought through a window in the interosseous membrane.
- A Pulvertaft weave is used for all tendon repairs.
- The tenodesis effect can be demonstrated immediately by flexing and extending the wrist and observing the finger motion (Fig. 26.11a, b).

Postoperative Management

- The patient can be discharged home on the day of surgery or the first postoperative day, depending on their general health and well-being and the adequacy of their pain control.
- At 2 weeks, the wound is inspected and a thermoplastic splint fashioned. This should protect the transfers. An outrigger may be used if the patient is cooperative.
- An experienced hand therapist should then commence a re-education program, stressing synergistic movements.
- After a further 4 weeks, this can be exchanged for a shorter thermoplastic splint which holds the wrist, fingers, and thumb in extension, but can be removed for exercise.
- Regular follow-up is advised either by the hand therapist or the hand surgeon, depending on what is locally available.

Flexor Carpi Ulnaris (FCU) Transfer

- The flexor carpi ulnaris can be used to motor the digital extensors instead of the flexor carpi radialis. Proximal muscle release is essential to gain adequate excursion and movement.
- This should not be used in posterior interosseous nerve palsy as it will augment the radial deviation of the wrist caused by the presence of a functioning extensor carpi radialis longus.
  - A longitudinal incision is made over the FCU with a transverse distal extension which allows access to the palmaris longus.
  - The FCU tendon is detached from the pisiform and traced proximally, stripping it from its muscular attachments if these persist distally.
  - An oblique incision is made over the dorso-ulnar aspect of the forearm.
  - The deep fascia overlying the flexor carpi ulnaris is excised, and the fascial attachments to the muscle belly are freed, allowing it to move freely.
  - The nerve supply to the flexor carpi ulnaris limits the proximal dissection entering 5 cm from its origin.
  - A subcutaneous tunnel is created around the ulnar border of the wrist through which the FCU tendon is passed.

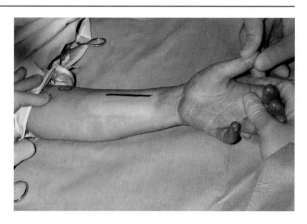

Fig. 26.12 A longitudinal incision is made on the radial aspect of the volar forearm

  - The line of pull from medial epicondyle to the extensor digitorum communis at the extensor retinaculum must be as straight as possible.
  - The FCU tendon is secured to all EDC tendons either end to end if the extensor digitorum communis are divided proximal to the extensor retinaculum or end to side if the extensor digitorum communis are left intact pending recovery.
  - The access to the dorsal forearm (extensor tendons) and pronator teres can be achieved with a chevron-type incision.

Postoperative Management

- The postoperative rehabilitation is similar to that where the flexor carpi radialis has been transferred.

Boyes Superficialis Transfer

- Pronator teres – extensor carpi radialis brevis / extensor carpi radialis longus.
- Flexor digitorum superficialis 4 – extensor digitorum communis 3, 4, 5.
- Flexor digitorum superficialis 3 – extensor indices proprius and extensor pollicis longus.
- Flexor carpi radialis – abductor pollicis longus.
  - A long incision is made on the volar aspect of the forearm down the radial side (Fig. 26.12).
  - The tendons of pronator teres, flexor digitorum superficialis to ring and middle fingers, and flexor carpi radialis are identified.

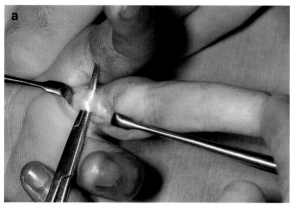

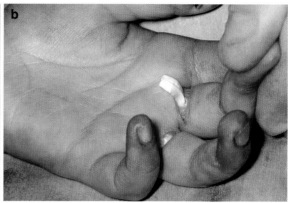

Fig. 26.13 (**a**) Through a transverse incision at the base of the finger, the tendon of the flexor digitorum superficialis to the ring and middlefingers are identified. This is achieved by confirming isolated movement of the proximal interphalangeal joint with traction on the tendon. (**b**) The tendon is cut proximal to the chiasm of Camper to prevent a swan-neck deformity of the proximal interphalangeal joint

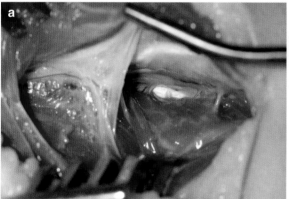

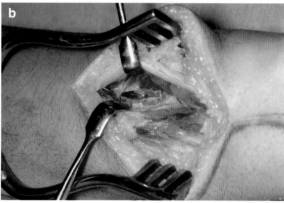

Fig. 26.14 (**a**) The anterior interosseous membrane is identified. The anterior interosseous neurovascular bundle is preserved while making a hole in the membrane for the flexor digitorum superficialis muscle belly to pass through. (**b**) A dorsal view showing the interosseous membrane and the posterior interosseous neurovascular bundle and the hole large enough to accommodate the muscle belly of the flexor digitorum superficialis for transfer to the extensor compartment

- The tendon of PT is dissected with a 3-cm strip of periosteum.
- The tendons of flexor digitorum superficialis are isolated by traction, confirming isolated movement of the pip joint (Fig. 26.13a).
- Short transverse incisions are made at the base of the middle and ring fingers and the flexor digitorum superficialis tendons divided proximal to Camper's chiasm (Fig. 26.13b).
- The divided flexor digitorum superficialis tendons are dissected proximally into the forearm to ensure adequate length for transfer through the interosseous membrane.
- A window is formed in the interosseous membrane proximally to allow transfer of the flexor tendons with preservation of the anterior and posterior interosseous neurovascular pedicles. The median nerve should also be protected (Fig. 26.14a, b).
- A second incision is made on the dorsum of the forearm.
- The tendons of extensor carpi radialis longus and brevis, extensor digitorum communis, and extensor pollicis longus are identified and dissected.
- The tendon and periosteal extension of the pronator teres are passed radially around the forearm in a subcutaneous plane above the

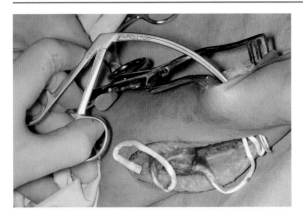

Fig. 26.15 The flexor digitorum tendon is passed smoothly through the interosseous membrane with the aid of the tendon passer

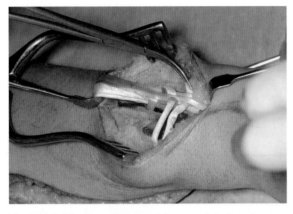

Fig. 26.16 The flexor digitorum 3 is woven into the extensor digitorum of the three ulnar digits

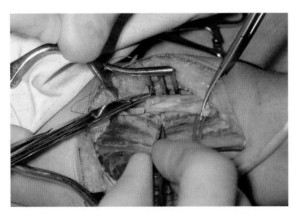

Fig. 26.17 A Pulvertaft weave is used to secure all tendon transfers

brachioradialis to be sutured to the extensor carpi radialis longus and brevis.

– The flexor digitorum superficialis tendons are passed through the interosseous membrane into the fourth dorsal compartment. Flexor digitorum superficialis to the middle finger is passed radially between flexor digitorum profundus and flexor pollicis longus, and the flexor digitorum superficialis of the ring finger is passed on the ulnar side to the flexor digitorum profundus (Fig. 26.15).

– Flexor digitorum superficialis of the middle finger is interwoven with the tendons of extensor indices and extensor pollicis longus, while flexor digitorum superficialis of the ring finger into extensor digitorum communis, leaving their proximal extensions intact (Fig. 26.16).

– The weave is completed under maximal tension with the fingers and thumb flexed into a fist.

– The flexor carpi radialis tendon is located through a short transverse radial wrist incision. This is then sutured to the abductor pollicis longus.

– Closure is performed of all wounds in two layers with absorbable sutures.

– The wounds are dressed.

– A plaster of Paris splint is fashioned to maintain the forearm in 15–30° of pronation, the wrist in 45° of extension, the metacarpophalangeal joints in 10–15° of flexion, and the thumb in maximal extension and abduction. The proximal interphalangeal joints can be left free.

Notes

• Alternatively, the flexor digitorum superficialis tendons can be rerouted through subcutaneous tunnels on the ulnar and radial borders of the forearm and wrist.

• The extensor retinaculum may be shortened if there is a risk of the tendon junctures impinging on its edge.

• A Pulvertaft weave is used for all tendon repairs (Fig. 26.17).

• When harvesting the flexor digitorum superficialis tendons, it is important to stay proximal to the chiasm to prevent laxity of the proximal interphalangeal joints and the occurrence of a swan-neck deformity.

Postoperative Management

- The patient can be discharged home on the day of surgery or the first postoperative day, depending on their general health and well-being and the adequacy of their pain control.
- At 2 weeks, the wound is inspected and a thermoplastic splint fashioned. This should protect the transfers. An outrigger may be used if the patient is cooperative.
- An experienced hand therapist should then commence a re-education program.
- After a further 4 weeks, this can be exchanged for a shorter thermoplastic splint which holds the wrist, fingers, and thumb in extension, but can be removed for exercise.

- Regular follow-up is advised either by the hand therapist or the hand surgeon, depending on what is locally available.
- Therapy should concentrate on voluntary control of flexor digitorum superficialis and not on the synergistic movements stressed in the FCU transfer.

Further Reading

Boyes JH. Tendon transfers for radial nerve palsy. Bull Hosp Jt Dis. 1960;21:97.

Green DP, Hotchkiss RN, Pederson WC, Wolfe SW. Green's operative hand surgery. 5th ed. New York: Churchill Livingstone; 2005.

Skoll PJ, Hudson DA, de Jager W, Singer M. Longterm results of tendon transfers for radial nerve palsy on patients with limited rehabilitation. Ann Plast Surg. 2000;45:122.

Tendon Transfers for Ulnar Nerve Palsy

27

Gráinne Bourke and Andrew Williams

Introduction

- Ulnar nerve injury impairs extrinsic and intrinsic hand movements along with sensory loss in the ulnar 1 and ½ digits and ulnar border of the hand.
- The loss of the intrinsic muscles in the hand results in severe impairment of fine motor actions including key pinch grip and fine precision movements. The loss of flexion of the little and ring distal interphalangeal joints combined with loss of the ulnar wrist flexor and loss of ulnar sensation impairs hand grasp and grip strength.
- There is a significant cosmetic defect with guttering between the metacarpals, flattening of the metacarpal arch and hypothenar eminence, and clawing of the metacarpophalangeal joints. This is paradoxically worse with functioning flexor digitorum profundi to the little and ring in low injuries or during the recovery phase in high lesions when these muscles have been reinnervated.
- Weak key pinch due to the loss of the first dorsal interosseous and thumb adductor is compensated for by interphalangeal joint flexion (flexor pollicis longus) and adduction (extensor pollicis longus). This is called Froment's sign.
- Ulnar clawing is due to the unopposed action of the extensor digitorum communis on the metacarpophalangeal joints leading to hyperextension of these joints and the flexion of the interphalangeal joints

by the long flexors. Normally, the intrinsic muscles would flex the metacarpophalangeal joint and extend the interphalangeal joints.
- The musculotendinous units affected in ulnar nerve palsy:
  – Low lesion:
      Adductor pollicis
      Deep head of flexor pollicis brevis
      Dorsal and palmar interossei
      Abductor digiti minimi, opponens digiti minimi, flexor digiti minimi
      Lumbricals to the ring and little fingers
  – High lesion as above plus:
      Flexor digitorum profundus to the little and ring finger
      Flexor carpi ulnaris

Indications

- Tendon transfers are used to provide active controlled motion where there is loss of function in the ulnar nerve distribution.
- Then aim of tendon transfers is to correct the claw deformity at the metacarpophalangeal joints and restore thumb stability and key pinch.

Timing of Tendon Transfers

- After failure of spontaneous nerve recovery or failure of recovery following nerve repair.
- As a substitute for nerve repair in those patients who are not suitable.

27

G. Bourke (✉) • A. Williams
Department of Plastic and Reconstructive Surgery,
Leeds Teaching Hospitals NHS Trust, Leeds, UK
e-mail: grainnebourke@nhs.net

Preoperative

Clinical Assessment

Signs of Ulnar Nerve Palsy
- Positive Froment's sign.
- Absent flexion of the DIP joints of the little and ring fingers.
- Claw deformity.
- Guttering between the metacarpals and flattening of the metacarpal arch.
- Weakness of wrist flexion.
- A tight first web space.
- Numbness of the ulnar side of the hand and the ulnar 1 and ½ digits.

Essential Requirements to Ensure a Good Functional Result
- Adequate soft tissue cover to enable tendon gliding.
- A stable underlying skeleton.
- Normal or near normal joint mobility of the wrist, fingers, and thumb.
- The musculotendinous units to be used for transfer are expendable and have adequate power and excursion.
- A cooperative and reliable patient.

Notes
- The extent and level of injury must be assessed. There may be anomalous innervation patterns. Up to 17% of individuals have median – ulnar connections in the distal forearm (Martin-Gruber connections).
- Key pinch relies upon thumb adduction, but also the stabilization of the index finger, through an abduction force.

Correction of the Claw Deformity

Static Procedures
- *Capsulodesis*
  - A palmer incision is made over the distal palmar crease.
  - The flexor tendons are retracted to expose the metacarpophalangeal joint capsule.
  - A transverse ellipse of palmer capsule is excised. The capsule is then resutured.
  - This should maintain 10–30° of metacarpophalangeal joint flexion when the digit extension is attempted.

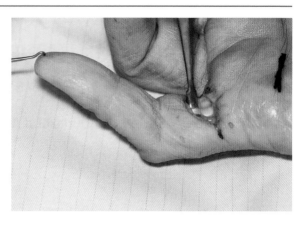

Fig. 27.1 The flexor digitorum superficialis is identified in the flexor sheath between the A1 and A2 pulleys

- *Bunnell's flexor pulley advancement* allows some bowstringing of the flexor tendons in the proximal finger.
- *Zancolli's fasciodermadesis* involves excision of palmar skin over the metacarpophalangeal joint and shortening of the pretendinous band of the palmar aponeurosis that causes flexion of the metacarpophalangeal joint.
- *Zancolli's metacarpophalangeal joint capsulodesis* involves releasing the A1 pulley and advancing the proximal edge of the volar plate onto the metacarpal neck. This yields about 20° of flexion of the metacarpophalangeal joint.

Note
- The results with static procedures are variable, and in most instances, the deformity recurs.
- This reconstruction does not influence the sequence of flexion in grip, and therefore, IPJ flexion is initiated prior to MCPJ flexion, in contrast to the normal sequence.
- If the patient is unable to actively extend the IPJs with the MCPJs passively flexed, a transfer should be considered which inserts onto the lateral bands of the extensor apparatus and will perform this action. Alternatively, if the extrinsic muscles can still perform this action, a transfer which addresses the MCPJ flexion deformity only needs to be considered.

Dynamic Procedures

- *Zancolli's lasso*
  - A volar incision is made to expose the flexor sheath over the A1 and A2 pulleys (Fig. 27.1).

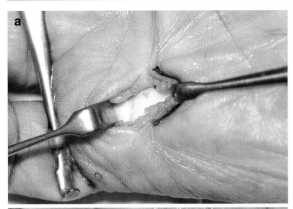

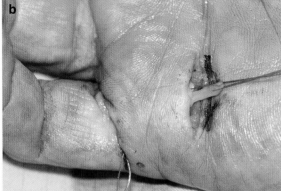

Fig. 27.2 (a) The proximal edge of the A1 pulley is identified. The flexor digitorum superficialis is identified within the sheath at this level. (b) It is divided and then passed over the A1 pulley proximally

- The FDS tendon is divided transversely between the A1 and A2 pulleys. It is important to confirm the flexor digitorum superficialis tendon by gentle traction which yields isolated proximal interphalangeal joint motion (Fig. 27.2a, b).
- It is passed over the A1 pulley from distal to proximal and sutured to itself with the MCPJ in 45° of flexion (Fig. 27.3).
- *Note*
  - Modifications have been described by Omer passing the tendon around the A2 pulley and by Anderson passing the tendon around both pulleys.
  - Usually the homodigital FDS is used, but the ring FDS can be split and used for correction of both the ring and little fingers.
  - In high lesions of the ulnar nerve, the flexor digitorum superficialis is the only ring and little finger flexor.

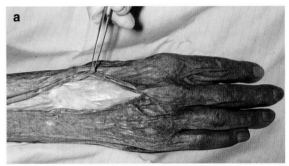

Fig. 27.3 The flexor digitorum is sutured to itself with a non-absorbable suture holding the metacarpophalangeal joint in flexion

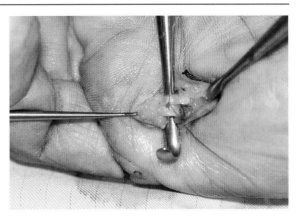

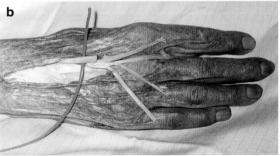

Fig. 27.4 (a) The extensor carpi radialis longus is harvested at the wristband mobilized proximally. (b) Illustrates the extension of the extensor carpi radialis longus with four digit slips. These are then passed either volar or dorsal through the lumbrical canal to be attached to the lateral band on the radial side of the 3 ulnar digits and on the ulnar side of the index finger

- *Brand procedures (Simultaneous MCPJ flexion and IPJ extension)*
  - A longitudinal incision is made on the dorsoradial aspect of the forearm to harvest the extensor carpi radialis longus/brevis tendon (Fig. 27.4a, b).

- The wrist extensor is then retrieved proximal to the extensor retinaculum.
- Sufficient tendon grafts are harvested to allow extension of the wrist extensor to the level of the lateral bands of the four fingers. This can be through a combination of plantaris/toe extensors or, alternatively, a segment of fascia lata that is split into four strands.
- A dorsoradial incision is made over the proximal phalanx of the ulnar 3 digits and a dorsoulnar incision over the index finger.
- A tendon retriever is passed along the lateral band proximally along the path of the lumbrical with the metacarpophalangeal joint flexed. The tendon retriever is then passed dorsally into proximal incision.
- Each division of the extended wrist extensor tendon is then passed via the tendon retriever into the appropriate lumbrical canal and to the lateral band.
- The tendon is secured with a non-absorbable suture.
- *Alternative volar route for Brand transfer*
  - The tendon of extensor carpi radialis longus or brevis is harvested and extended as previously described.
  - A transverse midpalmar incision is made.
  - A tendon retriever is passed proximally through the palmer incision into the carpal tunnel along the line of the flexor tendons.
  - The retriever is then passed radially and dorsally without tension and should exit through the dorsoradial incision beneath the brachioradialis.
  - The extended wrist extensor is then passed via the tendon retriever into the midpalmar incision.
  - A dorsoradial incision is made over the ulnar three fingers and dorsoulnar incision over the index finger.
  - The tendon retriever enables the passage of the tendon transfer along the route of the lumbrical with the metacarpophalangeal joint in flexion.
  - The transferred are sutured with the wrist neutral, the metacarpophalangeal joint flexed, and the interphalangeal joints extended.
- *Notes*
  - This technique was modified by Burkhalter by inserting the ECRL into the proximal phalanx and

by Brookes and Jones who used FCR and ECRL, inserted into A2 pulley of the affected digit.

Postoperative

- The hand is splinted with the wrist in neutral, the metacarpophalangeal joints flexed, and the interphalangeal joints extended for 4 weeks.
- At 4 weeks, this is replaced with a thermoplastic splint.
- A staged rehabilitation program is commenced under the care of a hand therapist.
- Regular review is essential to assess the progress and movement.

Tendon Transfers: Thumb Adduction

- *Flexor digitorum superficialis 3 or 4 to adductor pollicis (Littler)*
  - The flexor digitorum tendon is harvested proximal to Campers chiasm.
  - A palmer incision is made exposing the insertion of the adductor pollicis.
  - A tendon retriever aids the passage of the flexor tendon along a path deep to the other flexor tendons.
  - The tendon is sutured to insertion of adductor pollicis.
- *Brachioradialis transfer to adductor pollicis (Boyes)*
  - The brachioradialis tendon is harvested through a distal radial incision.
  - A tendon graft using either palmaris longus or plantaris is used to augment the transfer.
  - A palmer is made exposing the insertion of the adductor pollicis.
  - A tendon retriever is passed along the line of the adductor and then curved dorsally through the third intermetacarpal space.
  - The tendon transfer is then passed palmerly and inserted into the adductor insertion with a non-absorbable suture.
- *Notes*
  - Edgerton describes insertion onto the adductor tubercle.
  - In high ulnar nerve lesions, this transfer would result in an unacceptable loss of the ring and

little finger flexion due to the already impaired FDP function.
  – Smith and Omer describe techniques using the extensor carpi radialis brevis.

Tendon Transfers: Index Abduction

- *Abductor pollicis longus to first dorsal interosseous (Neviaser/Wilson)*
  – An incision is made at the base of the thumb over the abductor pollicis longus insertion.
  – The abductor pollicis longus has accessory slips which can be harvested for this transfer.
  – An incision is made on the radial side of the index finger over the base of the proximal phalanx.
  – A tendon graft is harvested (palmaris longus) and is used to extend the adductor tendon.
  – This is then tunnelled subcutaneously from the proximal to distal incisions and inserted into the radial lateral band of index and insertion of the first dorsal interosseous.
- *Extensor indices proprius to first dorsal interosseous (Bunnell)*
  – An incision is made over the index carpal to expose and harvest the extensor indices.
  – A transverse wrist incision is made, and the tendon is retrieved here to redirect it.
  – The tendon is then passed distally and sutured to a volar insertion on the metacarpal and the first dorsal interosseous insertion.
- *Notes*
  – The transfer of the extensor indices must be tight in order to achieve index finger stability.

- *Stabilization of the thumb*
  – Various methods of stabilizing the thumb using arthrodesis of either the metacarpophalangeal joint or the interphalangeal joint.
  – Tsuge has described a technique transferring part of the flexor pollicis longus to the extensor pollicis longus.

Further Reading

Blacker GJ, Lister GD, Kleinert HE. The abducted little finger in low ulnar nerve palsy. J Hand Surg. 1976;1:190.

Brand PW, Beach RB, Thompson DE. Relative tension and potential excursion of muscles in the forearm and hand. J Hand Surg. 1992;17:625.

Green DP, Hotchkiss RN, Pederson WC, Wolfe SW. Green's operative hand surgery. 5th ed. New York: Churchill Livingstone; 2005.

Hastings H, Davidson S. Tendon transfers for ulnar nerve palsy: evaluation of results and practical considerations. Hand Clin. 1988;4:167.

Neviaser RJ, Wilson JN, Gardner MM. Abductor pollicis longus transfer for replacement of the first dorsal interosseous. J Hand Surg. 1980;5:53.

Ozkan T, Ozer K, Gulgoren A. Three tendon transfer methods in reconstruction of ulnar nerve palsy. J Hand Surg. 2003; 28(1):35.

Smith RJ. Extensor carpi radialis brevis tendon transfer for thumb adduction: a study of power pinch. J Hand Surg. 1983;8:4.

Zancolli EA. Claw hand caused by paralysis of the intrinsic muscles: a simple surgical procedure for its correction. J Bone Joint Surg. 1957;39A:1076.

Surgical Technique of Anterior Cervical Discectomy and Fusion (ACDF)

28

Abhay S. Rao, Antony L.R. Michael, and Jake Timothy

Introduction

- ACDF has gained wide acceptance in the management of refractory symptoms attributed to cervical intervertebral disc disease.
- The aim of the procedure is to remove the intervertebral disc and variable amounts of bony osteophytes and the posterior longitudinal ligament (PLL) thus ensuring adequate decompression of the spinal cord and nerve roots.

Indications

- Spinal stenosis and compression of neural elements due to degeneration, trauma, and infection.
- Degenerative changes result in the formation of osteophytes which project posteriorly along with the PLL.
- Facet joint hypertrophy as well as infolding of the ligamentum flavum may contribute to the decrease in the dimensions of the spinal canal centrally and laterally.
- Trauma causing disc disruption is occasionally seen in facet joint subluxations and dislocations. In this situation, it is advisable to deal with the disc usually

with an ACDF prior to any posterior reduction and fixation.
- Infection causes compromise of the spinal canal by destruction and collapse of the vertebral body, epidural abscess formation, and occasionally posterior element involvement. This requires anterior debridement and fusion along with appropriate antibiotic therapy.
- In most cases, ACDF is done for complaints of predominantly radicular pain.

Preoperative Planning

Clinical Assessment

- It is important to obtain an adequate history specific to the presenting problem and general health with a view to determining the optimum treatment.
- General examination and spinal examination is important to determine and document the extent of impairment and fitness for surgery. Scoring systems such as the Neck Disability Index is useful to document the patient's condition preoperatively and postoperatively.
- Patients require satisfying the indications for surgery, and this varies from surgeon to surgeon.

Radiological Investigations

- These are carried out based on the patient history and examination findings.
- Hematological and biochemical investigations are tailored to patient requirements.

A.S. Rao (✉)
Department of Spinal Surgery,
Leeds Teaching Hospitals NHS Trust, Leeds, UK
e-mail: abhay.rao@leedsth.nhs.uk

A.L.R. Michael
Department of Trauma and Orthopaedics,
Leeds Teaching Hospitals NHS Trust, Leeds, UK

J. Timothy
Department of Neurosurgery, Leeds Teaching Hospitals
NHS Trust, Leeds, UK

- Plain radiographs are useful to show bony anatomy for preoperative planning and instability in flexion/extension views.
- CT scan is useful to give more bony detail; reconstructions in two and three dimensions often help to determine the pathology and surgical strategy.
- MRI scan is useful to see the neural elements and demonstrate soft tissue pathology.
- It is important to match radiological findings to patient symptoms and examination findings. If there is no good correlation, surgery may not be effective.

Operative Strategy

- The decision to perform discectomy with or without stabilization using instrumented fusion is determined on the basis of patient history, examination findings, and the results of the investigations.
- Occasionally two levels may have to be treated; rarely more than two levels require treatment, and in this situation, consideration needs to be given to a posterior procedure such as a skip laminectomy.
- Some surgeons would carry out ACDF without internal fixation. We prefer to internally fix the fusion level with plate in all cases of ACDF.
- The ACDF procedure may be carried from C2/3 to C7/T1.
- More proximal and distal levels are difficult in some cases due to patient anatomy.
- The more common levels are C4/5 and C5/6.

Anesthesia

- General anesthesia with a reinforced endotracheal tube.
- Hypotensive anesthesia within the limits tolerated by the patient reduces blood loss.
- Once the skin incision is marked, we infiltrate subdermally with local anesthetic and adrenaline (1:200000) to raise a wheal.

Patient Positioning and Equipment

- A conventional operating table is used.
- The anesthetized patient is brought into the operating theater on a trolley.

- The anesthetist guides the transfer of the patient onto the operating table.
- Patient is placed supine, and the head is supported with a horseshoe head support.
- The arms are supported on the sides. Calf pumps are always applied for intraoperative DVT prophylaxis; patient warming devices are used to prevent hypothermia.
- A rolled towel is placed at the level of the shoulder blades so that the patient's neck is optimally extended.
- Patient's shoulders should be pulled down with tape to allow intraoperative lateral radiography.
- Rarely, some in-line traction is required, and this is supplied by skull tongs with 5–10 lb of weight attached. It is important to release the traction force at the time of plating.
- Instruments required include: a standard dissection surgical set, self retaining blade retractors, upcutting instruments Kerrisons/Colcloughs, selection of PEEK (Poly ether ethyl ketone) cages, a cervical spine locking plate kit, high speed burr, and bone substitute of choice for facilitation of fusion.
- Real-time spinal cord monitoring using transcranial motor evoked and somatosensory evoked potential monitoring can be utilized to avoid potential neurological injury.

Incision

- Identify levels of proposed surgery and mark them using a marking pen. There are various ways of identifying the level. Several palpable anterior midline structures help. These include:
  1. Hard palate – arch of atlas
  2. Lower border of the mandible – C2/3
  3. Hyoid bone – C3
  4. Thyroid cartilage – C4/5
  5. Cricoid cartilage– C6
  6. Carotid (Chassaignac's) tubercle– C6
- In some cases, it is more reliable to mark the skin incision at the appropriate level with the aid of the image intensifier ensuring that the skin incision is centered on the appropriate level.
- A transverse incision is preferable (Fig. 28.1).
- Use the nearest skin crease as this gives a better scar.
- The operative field is prepared with a suitable antiseptic solution such as alcoholic iodine and draped with sterile drapes and an adhesive incision drape.

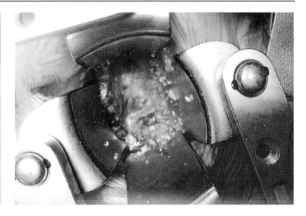

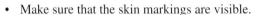

Fig. 28.1 Patient is placed supine. *Black dotted line* illustrates marking of transverse incision. *White dotted lines* represent borders of sternomastoid and thyroid cartilage

- Make sure that the skin markings are visible.
- We routinely use the right-sided approach though some surgeons would use the left-sided approach because of the theoretical reduction in risk of recurrent laryngeal nerve injury.

Surgical Exposure and Procedure

- Make an adequate skin incision with a scalpel and divide superficial fascia and platysma.
- The dissection plane is now in the internervous plane between the sternocleidomastoid and the strap muscles.
- The carotid sheath is then palpated and dissection carried out in the plane medial to the carotid sheath and lateral to the trachea/esophagus.
- This brings us to the prevertebral fascia which is dissected with sharp scissors/coagulating and cutting bipolar cautery.
- The plane is then between the right and left longus colli muscles which exposes the disc and adjacent vertebral bodies.
- At this stage, further radiographic confirmation of levels is obtained.
- Depending on the level of surgery the relationships will vary; a thorough knowledge of the anatomy of the region is required prior to embarking on this type of surgery.
- Once the longus colli have been identified, they are dissected to free the medial border under which the micro retractor of choice is placed thus protecting the soft tissues (Fig. 28.2).

Fig. 28.2 Placement of micro retractor for protection of the soft tissues is shown

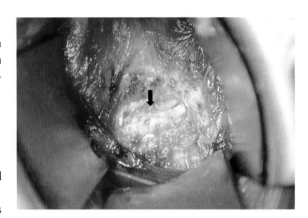

Fig. 28.3 *Arrow* demonstrates anterior annulus

- Right/left blades are often sufficient for single level surgery; however, further cranial and caudal blades may be placed to improve the size of the operative field.
- At this stage, we request the anesthetist to deflate and reinflate the cuff of the endotracheal tube and believe this reduces the stretch of the recurrent laryngeal nerve. Hemostasis is achieved and the discectomy is initiated.
- The anterior annulus is incised at the cephalic border of the caudal vertebra so that the lateral excursion of the blade is stopped by the uncovertebral joints avoiding injury to the vertebral artery (Fig. 28.3).
- The blade is turned superiorly up to the cephalad vertebra and then again turned to the midline thus removing a rectangular piece of the annulus.

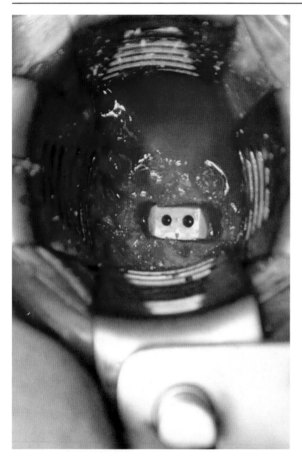

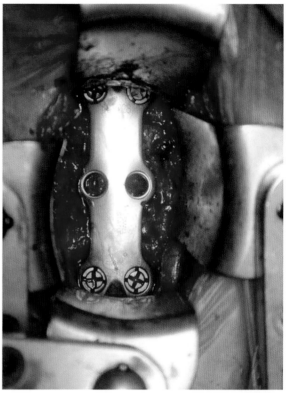

Fig. 28.5 Implantation of cervical spine locking plate is shown fixed to the adjacent vertebral bodies with two locking screws in each vertebral body

Fig. 28.4 The correct size cage chosen is shown in situ with packed bone substitute of choice

- The disc is then removed with curettes and pituitary forceps. We use a burr to remove the overhang from the cephalad vertebra and to create a rectangular space to work.
- It is important to ensure that the bony end plate is not breached and that the cartilaginous end plate is completely removed.
- Any anterior osteophytes are removed with the burr to allow us to determine the anterior vertebral anatomy. This is important to ensure correct placement of the plate.
- The burr is used to go posteriorly up to the PLL. Once the PLL is reached, a dissecting hook is used to go through the PLL into the epidural space.
- Once the epidural space is entered, upcutting instruments (Kerrisons/Colcloughs) with thin cervical foot plates are used to excise the discoligamentous structures compressing the neural elements.

- Once there is adequate decompression of the spinal cord and nerve roots, we select the intervertebral cage to be used by sizing with trials.
- We prefer a PEEK (Poly ether ethyl ketone) cage with a lordotic shape to restore normal cervical lordosis.
- The correct size cage is then packed with bone substitute of choice and inserted with gentle tapping (Fig. 28.4).
- Once the cage is satisfactorily in place, it is important to remove the weight attached to the traction tongs.
- The plate of choice is then sized and contoured. We use a cervical spine locking plate. This is fixed to the adjacent vertebral bodies with two locking screws in each vertebral body (Fig. 28.5).
- The screw length is determined by measuring from preoperative radiographs and from a depth gauge measuring device intraoperatively.
- The retractors are removed, hemostasis achieved, and a suction drain placed to prevent postoperative hematoma.

Closure

- The wound is closed in layers with platysma in one layer and subcuticular closure of skin.
- Transverse steristrips and a waterproof dressing are then applied.
- Remove the traction tongs.

Postoperative Care

- After wound dressing, move patient carefully to the trolley.
- The anesthesia is reversed and the drain opened.
- An operation note is made with details of the operation, details on implants used if any, and postoperative instructions.
- Monitor the neurological status frequently, every 15 min for 2 h, every 30 min for 2 h, and every hour for 2 h; if after the 6 h there is no cause for concern, it is repeated 4 hourly.
- Patients are usually able to return to a spine ward from the recovery ward.
- Patients are usually mobilized later on the same day or on the first postoperative day by the physiotherapists.
- Check radiographs and blood tests are done and the drain removed at 24–48 h depending on drainage.

Rehabilitation/Follow-up

- Discharge patients when they are independently mobile.
- Keep the wound dry for 7 days.
- Arrange outpatient physiotherapy.
- Review patients in the outpatient clinic at approximately 6 weeks, 3 months, and 6 months. Obtain radiographs to ensure satisfactory progress.

Further Reading

Bohlman HH, Emery SE, Goodfellow DB, Jones PK. Robinson anterior cervical discectomy and arthrodesis for cervical radiculopathy: long-term follow-up of one hundred and twenty-two patients. J Bone Surg (Am). 1993;75:1298–307.

Hilibrand AS, Fye MA, Emery SE, Palumbo MA, Bohlman HH. Increased rate of arthrodesis with strut grafting after multi-level anterior cervical decompression. Spine. 2002;27:146–51.

Chang SW, Kakarla UK, Maughan PH, DeSanto J, Fox D, Theodore N, et al. Four-level anterior cervical discectomy and fusion with plate fixation: radiographic and clinical results. Neurosurgery. 2010;66(4):639–46.

Microdiscectomy/ Microdecompression for Intraspinal Intervertebral Disc Prolapses and Lateral Recess Stenosis

Robert A. Dunsmuir

Indications

- Microdiscectomy/microdecompressionis suitable for leg pain/sciatica caused by the following conditions:
  - Cauda equina syndrome secondary to prolapsed intervertebral discs
  - Sciatica (leg pain) with leg muscle weakness (e.g., foot drop) or without secondary to prolapsed intervertebral discs
  - Sciatica (leg pain) secondary to lateral recess stenosis
  - Sciatica (leg pain) due to synovial facet joint cysts

Preoperative Planning

Clinical Assessment

- Patients usually present with leg pain in a dermatomal distribution of one or more nerve roots.
- Symptoms could be suggestive of cauda equina syndrome or nerve root irritation on femoral nerve stretching or sciatic nerve stretching.
- Signs of muscle weakness in a particular muscle group may be present (e.g., partial foot drop suggestive of an L5 root lesion).

R.A. Dunsmuir
Department of Trauma and Orthopaedic Surgery,
Leeds Teaching Hospitals NHS Trust,
Leeds, UK
e-mail: robert.dunsmuir@leedsth.nhs.uk

- Absence of knee or ankle reflexes may be present, and this is typically unilateral but can be bilateral in cauda equina syndrome.
- Rectal examination for perianal sensation, anal tone, and squeeze is mandatory if there are any symptoms that may suggest cauda equina syndrome.

Radiological Assessment

- The gold standard for identification of a disc prolapse is MRI scanning (Fig. 29.1). Gadolinium can be injected to look for epidural fibrosis if the patient has had previous surgery.
- If MRI scan cannot be tolerated or if patient has metallic implant, e.g., a cardiac pacemaker, then a CT scan or CT myelogram can be performed.

Classification

- Disc prolapse can be classified by the degree of prolapse or the position of the prolapse within the spinal canal:
  Degree of prolapse
    Protruded
    Extruded
    Sequestrated
  Position of prolapse
    Central
    Sub-articular
    Foraminal
    Extra-foraminal

Fig. 29.1 Axial T2 MRI showing extruded prolapsed intervertebral disc

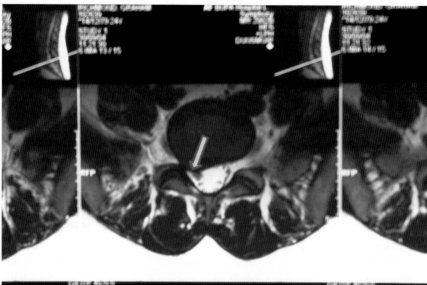

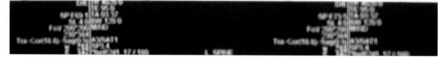

Operative Treatment

Anesthesia

- Patients are operated on under general anesthesia.
- As the patient will be "prone" throughout the procedure, it is necessary to use endotracheal intubation with an armored endotracheal tube.

Operating Microscope

- The eyepieces of the operating microscope are adjusted for the surgeon and the assistant before the operation starts. The microscope can then be draped with its sterile microscope drape.
- The operating microscope gives the surgeon the advantage of illumination and magnification, making the procedure safer for the patient.
- Similar goals can be achieved using mini-open approaches such as the one described here with the aid of endoscopes attached to frames.
- Some surgeons use headlamps without any aid to magnify the wound. The author believes this method to be an inferior method of surgery to the method described in this chapter.

Patient Positioning

- Microdiscectomy can be performed with the patient in two positions – knee/chest position or prone on a spinal frame.
- Either position is used to attempt to maximally flex the spinal segment being operated on.
- These maneuvers aim to stretch the ligamentum flavum and make its resection easier.

Knee/Chest Position (Fig. 29.2a–c)

- The patient is brought into the operating theater on a trolley.
- The anesthetist guides the transfer of the patient onto the operating table while protecting the head and neck position.
- The patient is rolled prone onto the operating table. The patient support onto which they "sit" is positioned (Fig. 29.2a).
- The patient is lifted into position. This requires a minimum of five people. The anesthetist controls the head and neck. Each shoulder is lifted by one person who lifts the patient by putting their hand onto the patient's anterior chest wall just anterior to the shoulder. The

surgeon lifts the pelvis. A further person pushes the patient's legs under the pelvis as it is lifted. As a result, knees and hips are flexed to 90°. These simultaneous movements lift the patient into position.

- The patient's bottom is then rested onto the support. Pillows or a chest support put under the patient's chest, and the patient rests on these (Fig. 29.2b). The patient's face rests in a "Prone View" (Fig. 29.2c).
- The position of the tabletop is changed to bring the lumbar spine parallel to the floor (Fig. 29.2a).
  Precautions
      Ensure there is no pressure on the patient's axillae.
      Ensure that the patient's feet are free and not overextended at the ankle.
      Ensure the patient's eyes are visible using the "Prone View."
      Ensure no pressure is applied to abdomen and its contents. This will minimize back pressure from abdominal veins anastomosing with epidural veins.
  Potential problems
      Pressure problems on skin of chest and knees
      Brachial plexus stretching
      Pressure on eye

Prone on Frame (Fig. 29.3)

- A "Wilson Frame" is used for prone spinal operations.
- The patient is brought into the operating theater on a trolley.
- The anesthetist guides the transfer of the patient onto the operating table.
- The patient is rolled prone onto the operating table on top of the Wilson Frame. The patient's head is rested in the Prone View.
- The Wilson Frame is flexed into its maximum position.
  Precautions
      Ensure there is no pressure on the patient's axillae.
      Ensure that the patient's knees and ankles are not overextended.
      Ensure the patient's eyes are visible using the "Prone View" especially after the frame has been flexed up to its maximum position. The patient

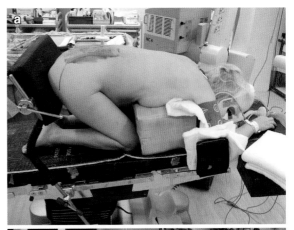
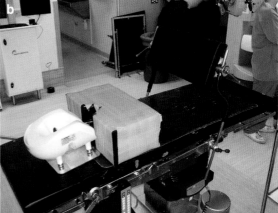
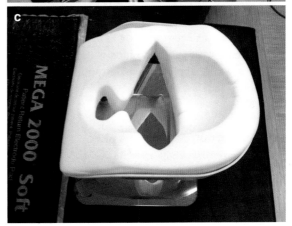

Fig. 29.2 (**a**) The knee/chest position showing the patient's bottom and chest supported on rests. The lumbar spine at the level to be operated on is parallel to the floor. (**b**) The supports used for the knee/chest position. (**c**) The "Prone View." This device allows the patient's eyes to be seen throughout the operation, and the memory foam protects the bony prominences of the face

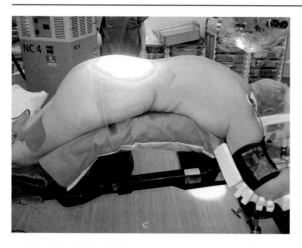

Fig. 29.3 Patient lying prone on the Wilson Frame which is flexed to its maximum position

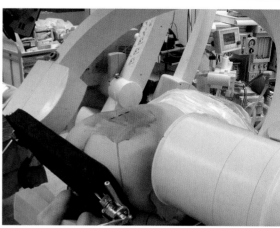

Fig. 29.4 Checking the correct operative level using the image intensifier to locate the epidural needle

can "slip" distally during this procedure, and pressure can be applied to the orbits.

Ensure no pressure is applied to abdomen and its contents. This will minimize back pressure from abdominal veins anastomosing with epidural veins.

Potential problems

Pressure problems on skin of chest, flanks, and knees

Brachial plexus stretching

Pressure on eyes

- No matter what patient position is used, calf pumps are always applied for intraoperative DVT prophylaxis.

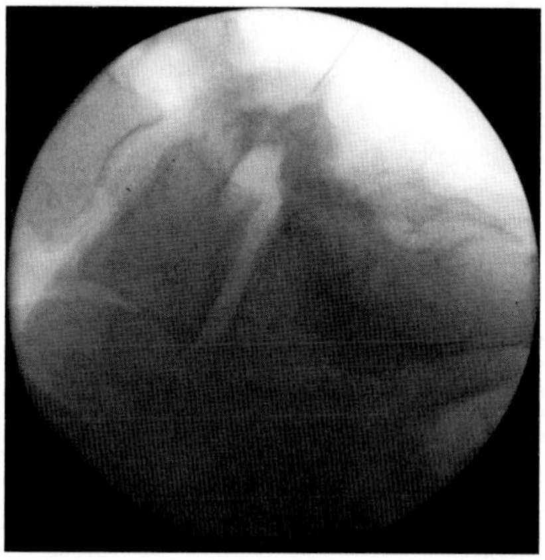

Level Checking

- The image intensifier is used to identify the correct operative level.
- The palpable spinous processes are marked with a permanent marker pen.
- The skin is prepared with alcoholic chlorhexidine or Betadine solutions.
- An epidural needle is pushed through the skin perpendicular to the skin surface. The needle is passed through the soft tissue until near the spinal column (Fig. 29.4).
- An x-ray image is obtained. This will determine if the selected level is over the disc space to be operated upon. If the needle is not correctly positioned, remove

Fig. 29.5 Image intensifier view showing the epidural needle pointing to the disc level to be operated on

the needle and reinsert it more proximally or distally as directed by the original needle position.

- Repeat this until you are happy that the needle is directly over the correct disc space (Fig. 29.5).
- In the knee/chest position, the image intensifier needs to come over the top of the patient to get a lateral view (Fig. 29.4). If using a frame the image intensifier can come over the top of the patient, or if the operating table allows, go under the table to get a lateral view (Fig. 29.6).
- Once the correct disc level is identified, this level is marked with two skin marks at 90° to the long axis of the spinal column at the level of the disc, and the upper and lower extents of the skin incision are marked (Fig. 29.7).

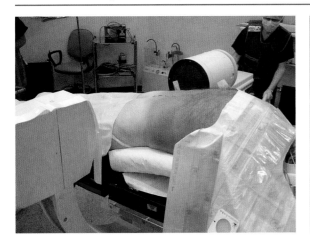

Fig. 29.6 Checking the level using the image intensifier under the table

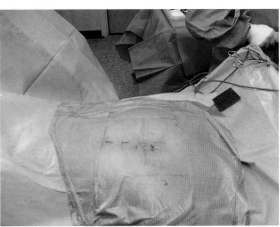

Fig. 29.8 The patient draped showing the skin markings for the spinous processes, level of the disc, and the extent of the skin incision

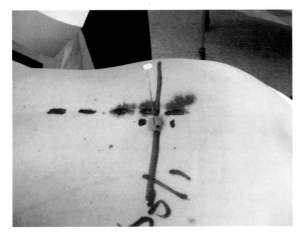

Fig. 29.7 The spinous processes are marked. A line is drawn perpendicular to the long axis of the spine over the place where the epidural needle was placed. The extent of the skin incision is marked

Draping

- The skin is prepped with the antiseptic solution of choice.
- Adhesive paper drapes are applied and the operative field covered with an occlusive dressing (e.g., Opsite) (Fig. 29.8).

Surgical Exposure

- The skin incision 2–3 cm in length is made over the predetermined level.

- Divide superficial and deep fascia in line with the skin incision until the thoracolumbar fascia is identified.
- Make a C-shaped incision (base toward the spinous processes) from the upper edge of the spinous process above the operative level to the lower edge of the spinous process below the operative level.
- The thoracolumbar fascia is in two layers at the lower lumbar spine, and care should be taken to ensure both layers are divided.
- Separate thoracolumbar fascia from the attached erector spinae muscles by blunt dissection using a Cobb retractor.
- Apply a stay suture to the apex of the "C" of the fascia. An artery forceps is applied to this suture, and the fascia is retracted using this suture by laying the forceps over the opposite side of the patient from where the surgeon is standing.
- Using two Cobb retractors, detach the erector spinae muscles from the spinous processes above and below the disc level that is being operated upon and from the interspinous ligament between these spinous processes. Note: in this area, there is frequently found a small multifidus tendon which will not divide by blunt dissection and often requires diathermy to divide it.
- At this point, the muscles are retracted toward the surgeon, and a muscle retractor of the required depth is inserted (Fig. 29.9a).
- The retractor is opened to allow visualization of both laminae. A third retractor is inserted to triangulate the retraction (Fig. 29.9b, c).

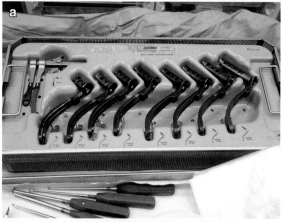

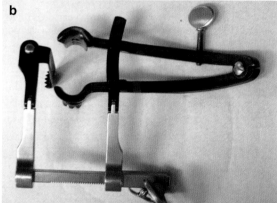

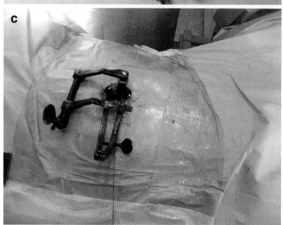

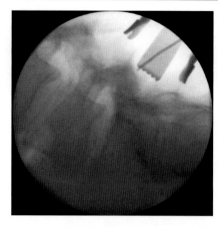

Fig. 29.10 Image intensifier view showing the retractor under the lower edge of the proximal lamina

Fig. 29.9 (**a**) Visualization of muscle retractors. These are of different lengths to allow for different depths of wounds. (**b**) The retractor fitted illustrating how the three blades provide retraction. (**c**) Retractor in situ (viewed from the assistant's side of the table)

- This will give a good view of both laminae and the ligamentum flavum. At this point, before any tissue is divided or resected, it is wise to recheck that you

are at the correct level using the image intensifier (Fig. 29.10).

- A Watson Chain retractor is placed under the lower edge of the proximal lamina of the spinal level to be opened.
- The operating microscope is brought into the operative field, having had a specialist sterile drape applied.
- The ligamentum flavum is divided transversely to divide the fibers. A "Mercedes Benz" type incision is employed as it allows the flavum fibers to retract more easily when divided (Fig. 29.11a). This incision is deepened until the epidural fat is identified.
- The hole through which this fat is seen is enlarged using a Watson Chain retractor.
- Through this hole, a Colcloughs dissector (2 mm or 3 mm) is inserted (Fig. 29.11b).
- Excise the flavum and the adjacent edges of the laminae. Open the canal sufficiently laterally to see the edge of the dural sac and the shoulder of the nerve root (Fig. 29.12). This usually requires undercutting of the facet joint and in so doing gives a good posterior decompression of the nerve root.
- If microdecompression only is being performed, it is mandatory to ensure that the facet is resected sufficiently to free the nerve root and the nerve root canal is freed of obstructions.
- The edge of the dural sac is gently retracted medially using a "Swedish retractor" or a Watson Chain retractor (Fig. 29.13). This exposes the disc prolapse or sequestrated fragment.
- Remove any loose disc fragments with pituitary forceps. If the annulus is intact, insert an epidural

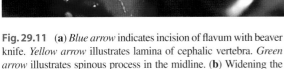

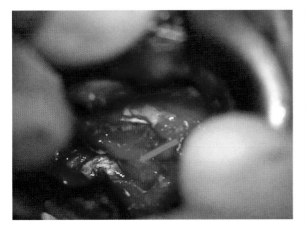

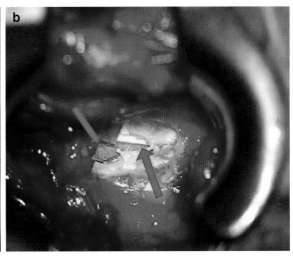

Fig. 29.11   (**a**) *Blue arrow* indicates incision of flavum with beaver knife. *Yellow arrow* illustrates lamina of cephalic vertebra. *Green arrow* illustrates spinous process in the midline. (**b**) Widening the hole in the ligamentum flavum with a Kerrison rongeur. *Blue arrow* illustrates dural sac. *Green arrow* illustrates medial edge of incised flavum defect

Fig. 29.12   The exposed dural sac and nerve root after resecting the ligamentum flavum and adjacent edges of the laminae. *Blue arrow* indicates nerve root branching off the dural sac

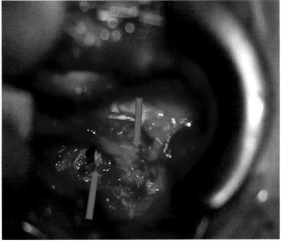

Fig. 29.13   *Blue arrow* illustrates nerve root. *Green arrow* illustrates prolapsed intervertebral disc

needle into the disc and recheck the level using the image intensifier (Fig. 29.14).

- Once it has been confirmed that the needle is in the correct disc, make a cruciate incision in the annulus (no. 15 blade – Swann Morton, ensuring sharp edge faces away from dura).
- The disc space is emptied of nuclear material using pituitary forceps.
- When the disc is cleared of nuclear material, the nerve root retractor is removed. The nerve root is now decompressed (Fig. 29.15).

Closure

- Ensure that hemostasis is achieved before removing the muscle retractors.
- This minimizes the risk of postoperative hematoma formation and subsequent neurological compromise.
- The anesthetist can be asked to perform a Valsalva procedure on the patient in order to look for any signs of CSF leak.

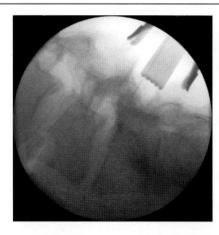

Fig. 29.14 Image intensifier view of epidural needle in the disc to be operated on

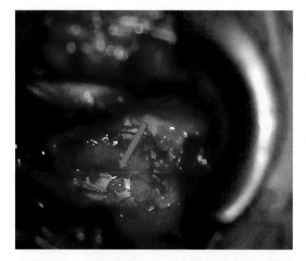

Fig. 29.15 *Blue arrow* illustrates the decompressed nerve root

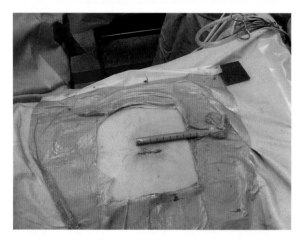

Fig. 29.16 The final sutured wound

- Remove the muscle retractors and close the wound in layers:
  1 Vicryl, J-shaped needle to reconstruct thoracolumbar fascia
  2.0 PDS/Vicryl to subcutaneous tissues
  Absorbable subcuticular suture to the skin (Fig. 29.16)
- Infiltrate the wound with Marcain 0.5%.
- Apply steristrips transversely over the wound and apply a dressing.

Postoperative Observations

- On return to the ward, patients are allowed to mobilize as pain permits.
- Neurological observations and cauda equina observations are performed:
  Every 15 min for 2 h
  Every 30 min for 2 h
  Every hour for 2 h
- If all is well at this stage, these observations are performed 4 hourly thereafter.

Rehabilitation

- When the patient is freely mobile and is voiding normally, they are discharged (normally the day following surgery).
- Lifting and strenuous exercises of lumbar spine are discouraged for 6 weeks.

Outpatient Follow-up

- Patients are routinely reviewed 6 weeks after surgery, and physiotherapy is organized as required.
- Patient is discharged to the care of the General Practitioner thereafter.

Further Reading

Dunsmuir RA. Prolapsed Intervertebral Discs. Curr Orthop. 2005;18:434–40.
Farndon DF, Milette PC. Nomenclature and Classification of Lumbar Disc Pathology. Spine. 2001;26:E93–113.
Caspar W. A new Surgical procedure for lumbar disc herniation causing less tissue damage through a microsurgical approach. Adv Neurosurg. 1977;4:74–80.

Lumbar Decompression and Instrumented Fusion

30

Robert A. Dunsmuir and Antony L.R. Michael

Introduction

- Laminectomy is the removal of the lamina of the vertebra for purposes of decompression of the spinal canal.
- It is combined with variable amounts of bone removal from the posterior elements such as the facet joints to adequately decompress the thecal sac and the nerve roots.
- The ligamentum flavum which runs from the anterior aspect of the cephalad lamina to the superior aspect of the caudal lamina is also usually resected.
- Laminectomy may be done at one or more levels. It is combined with instrumented posterolateral fusion in cases where there is instability of the spinal column as a result of the pathology being treated or where instability will be produced due to the amount of bone that needs to be removed for adequate decompression.

Indications

- Lumbar decompression with instrumented fusion is suitable for leg pain/sciatica due to neurogenic claudication (central canal stenosis, lateral recess stenosis, spondylolisthesis, and discogenic disk disease).

R.A. Dunsmuir (✉)
Department of Trauma and Orthopaedic Surgery,
Leeds Teaching Hospitals NHS Trust,
Leeds, UK
e-mail: robert.dunsmuir@leedsth.nhs.uk

A.L.R. Michael
Department of Trauma and Orthopaedics,
Leeds Teaching Hospitals NHS Trust,
Leeds, UK

- The "stenotic" effect could be related with a variety of potential etiologies, such as:

Congenital or developmental causes.

Degeneration: Degenerative changes result in facet joint hypertrophy, infolding of the ligamentum flavum, and posterior bulging of the intervertebral disk; all contributing to the decrease in the dimensions of the spinal canal centrally and laterally.

Tumor: Tumor, most commonly metastatic, can cause stenosis by bulging of the vertebral body posteriorly, expansion of the pedicles medially, and posterior elements anteriorly.

Trauma: Fracture of the vertebral body, pedicles, and posterior elements may cause compromise of the spinal canal.

Infection: Infection causes compromise of the spinal canal by destruction and collapse of the vertebral body, epidural abscess formation, and occasionally posterior element involvement.

Preoperative Planning

Clinical Assessment

- Presence of leg pains when walking (neurogenic claudication).
- Patients also described numbness, heaviness, and clumsiness of the lower limbs attributes to walking.
- Stopping walking eases the symptoms.
- Symptoms of bladder and bowel dysfunction do occur but frequently occur later.
- Neurological examination of the lower limbs is commonly normal.

P.V. Giannoudis (ed.), *Practical Procedures in Elective Orthopaedic Surgery*,
DOI 10.1007/978-0-85729-820-1_30, © Springer-Verlag London Limited 2012

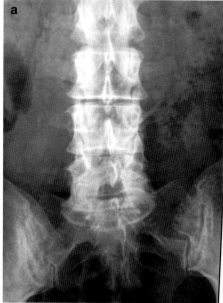
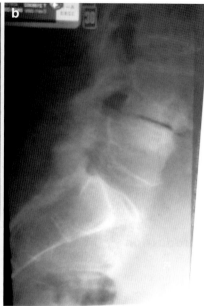

Fig. 30.1 (**a**) AP X-ray of the lumbar spine showing marked degenerative changes. (**b**) Lateral X-ray of the lumbar spine showing degenerate L4/5 spondylolisthesis and a grade one slip

- Peripheral pulses should always be checked. Impalpable pulse may *indicate vascular claudication.*
- In the presence of bladder and bowel symptoms, a rectal examination is mandatory. – *Possible cauda equina syndrome.*

Investigations

- Hematological and biochemical investigations are tailored to patient requirements.
- Plain radiographs are useful to show bony anatomy for preoperative planning and instability in flexion/extension views (Fig. 30.1a, b).
- If a spondylolisthesis is present, these films can be used to determine the degree of slip.
- CT scan is useful to give more bony detail; reconstructions in two and three dimensions often help to determine the pathology and surgical strategy.
- CT myelogram can be used when the patient is unable to have an MRI scan and can often give very precise information regarding the soft tissue compression on the neural structures.
- MRI scan is useful to see the neural elements and demonstrates soft tissue pathology as well as giving a more accurate assessment of the degree of stenosis (Fig. 30.2). Recent advances in upright MRI have the potential to demonstrate dynamic stenosis and instability.

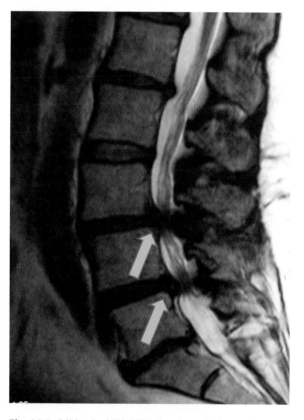

Fig. 30.2 Midsagittal T2 MRI showing spinal stenosis at the L3/4 and L4/5 disk spaces

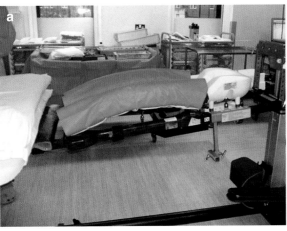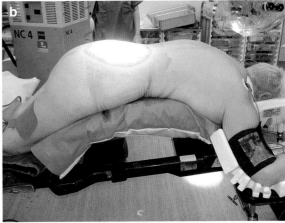

Fig. 30.3 (**a**) The OSI table with a Wilson Frame attachment. This allows circumferential X-ray imaging of the spine, should pedicle screw insertion be required. (**b**) Patient lying on Wilson Frame with the frame arched to maximum

- Isotope bone scan is used if metastatic disease is suspected as the cause of stenosis. This will show the extent of metastatic disease and can help in determining what operative intervention is possible.

Operative Strategy

- The decision to decompress OR decompress and stabilse with instrumented fusion and number of levels to be treated is determined on the basis of patient history, examination findings, and the results of the investigations.
- Laminectomy and undercutting facetectomy are adequate in patients with degenerative spinal stenosis without instability.
- Instrumented posterolateral fusion is done where there is preoperative instability, e.g., spondylolisthesis or when instability will be produced as a result of the amount of bone removed for adequate decompression.

Anesthesia

- General anesthesia with a reinforced endotracheal tube is the norm.
- Hypotensive anesthesia within the limits tolerated by the patient reduces blood loss.
- In cases of multilevel decompression, instrumented fusion, etc., intra-operative red cell salvage is used.
- The use of muscle relaxants aids surgical dissection and retraction.

Patient Positioning

- Use a spinal table which allows circumferential radiographic access (OSI). A spinal frame such as the "Wilson Frame" is used (Fig. 30.3a).
- The patient is brought into the operating theater on a trolley. The anesthetist guides the transfer of the patient onto the operating table. The patient is rolled prone onto the operating table on top of the Wilson Frame (Fig. 30.3b).
- The patient's head is rested in the "Prone View" that molds to the face and allows visualization of the patient's eyes ensuring there is no pressure.
- The Wilson Frame is flexed into its maximum position to flex the spine which will open up the interlaminar interval allowing easier access to the epidural space.

Tip: It is important to flatten the Wilson Frame prior to the application of rods and final tightening to ensure optimum sagittal contour.

Precautions

- Ensure there is no pressure on the patient's axillae, and the shoulders are not over abducted.
- Ensure that the patient's knees are flexed, and ankles are not over extended.
- Ensure the patients eyes are visible using the "Prone View" especially after the frame has been flexed up to its maximum position. The patient can "slip" distally during this procedure, and pressure can be applied to the orbits.

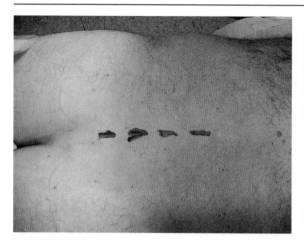

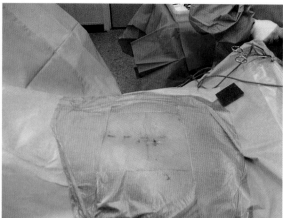

Fig. 30.4 Skin marked over the spinous processes in the operative field. The center of the operative field can be marked by lying a metal rod on the skin and localizing the correct level using the image intensifier. Alternatively, a spinal needle inserted into the skin can be used to localize the correct operative level

Fig. 30.5 Sterile drapes and occlusive dressing applied allowing visualization of skin markings

- Ensure no pressure applied to abdomen and its contents. This will minimize back pressure from abdominal veins anastomosing with epidural veins and thus reduce intraoperative bleeding.
- Calf pumps are always applied for intraoperative DVT prophylaxis; patient warming devices are used to prevent hypothermia.

Planning the Incision

- Mark levels of proposed surgery on the skin with permanent marker with the use of the image intensifier. This will ensure that the skin incision is of adequate length and centered on the appropriate level (Fig. 30.4).

Draping

- The operative field is prepared with a suitable antiseptic solution such as alcoholic iodine or chlorhexidine and draped with sterile drapes. An adhesive incision drape is applied to the exposed skin ensuring that the skin markings are visible (Fig. 30.5).

Surgical Exposure and Procedure

- A posterior midline skin incision of adequate length is made. The skin incision is made with a scalpel;

superficial and deep fasciae are divided with cutting cautery.
- Bilateral dissection of the paraspinal muscles is carried in the subperiosteal plane with the help of Cobb Elevators and diathermy ensuring minimal devitalization of tissues.
- The dissection is carried laterally up to the level of the facet joints in the case of a simple laminectomy.
- The dissection is taken to the tip of the transverse processes for instrumented fusion (Fig. 30.6).
- It is important to preserve the facet joint capsules till the definitive levels of fusion are determined by further intraoperative radiographs.
- Adequate self-retaining retractors are used to keep the operative field exposed.
- The lamina/laminae to be removed are identified using the image intensifier.
- The spinous process of the vertebra having the laminectomy is excised.
- The midline gap between the two halves of the ligamentum flavum is found, and this gap developed using a Watson Cheyne Dissector. Once the epidural space is identified, the ligamentum flavum can be excised using Colclough/Kerrison up cutters.
- This gap is often very difficult to find. In these circumstances, the midline junction of the laminae can be resected superiorly using Kerrison up cutters.
- This resection is extended proximally until the superior edge of the lamina is excised. This creates a central trough in the lamina.
- The flavum and lamina is then excised laterally on both sides with rongeurs. In the case of laminectomy, it is important to preserve the integrity of

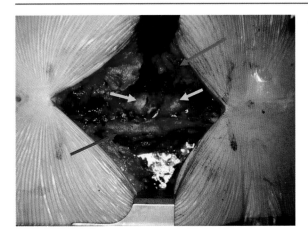

Fig. 30.6 The posterior aspect of the vertebrae exposed to show the tips of the laminae. *Blue arrow* illustrates spinous processes interconnected with supraspinous ligament. *Green arrow* illustrates the paraspinal muscles subperiosteally elevated and mobilized laterally. *Yellow arrows* illustrate the superior and inferior left sided facet joints following preparation with the Cobb Elevator

the facet joints and the pars interarticularis. This prevents destabilization of the spinal level being decompressed.

- The nerve roots are identified and decompressed laterally by removing the osteophytes and hypertrophied joint capsule from the undersurface of the facets.
- For the instrumented fusion, the pedicle screws are inserted via standard technique.
- Pedicle screw insertion can be performed before or after decompression of the dural sac. Pedicle entry points can be identified using the transverse process, pars, and facet joint as landmarks. Pedicle markers are then placed and biplanar imaging obtained.
- If the entry points are satisfactory, the pedicle probe is introduced to create a track for the screw to be inserted.
- Before placing the screw, each screw hole is examined with a blunt-end probe to check for bony integrity of the pedicle.
- The length of the screw is measured from the pedicle awl and the diameter determined from the dimensions of the pedicle. The appropriate pedicle screw is then inserted under radiographic guidance to ensure optimum placement.
- The transverse processes are decorticated and the posterolateral gutter prepared by removal of soft tissue until the intertransverse fascia is seen thus providing a good bed for the bone graft.

- Once adequate decompression is achieved, *the Wilson Frame is lowered;* precontoured rods or rods contoured to the optimum sagittal profile are then selected, length checked, placed, and tightened on to the pedicle screws.
- Distraction between the pedicle screws is applied for indirect foraminal decompression if required before final tightening of the rod screw construct.
- The bone graft is harvested from the posterior iliac crest and used in isolation or mixed with bone substitute and local bone obtained from the decompression (all soft tissue removed). This is placed in the posterolateral gutter extending between the transverse processes of the levels to be fused (Fig. 30.7).
- In cases of lateral recess stenosis, it is important to carry the decompression of the nerve out beyond the lateral recess. This may require excision of the inferior facet and pars interarticularis on that side (Fig. 30.8).
- Hemostasis is achieved, and a Valsalva maneuver carried out to ensure there is no leak of CSF.
- The retractors are removed, and a suction drain placed to prevent postoperative epidural hematoma.

Special Note.

For a 360° fusion, a cage, it is necessary to be inserted in the intervertebral disk space. For those conditions, discectomy must be performed, and vertebral end plates have to be decorticated. Following that, the cage (PEEK, stainless steel, tantalum or other, or tricortical bone allograft) is inserted in the intervertebral space with (usually) or without bone graft. There are various techniques with which the cage could be applied – *ALIF* Anterior Lumbar Interbody Fusion, – *PLIF* Posterolateral, Lumbar Interbody Fusion, – *TLIF* Transforaminal Lumbar Interbody Fusion, and – *XLIF* Extreme Lateral Lumbar Interbody Fusion.

Closure

- Drain is recommended for multilevel decompression – fusion, but it is rarely in use for a single level operation. In addition, it is not advisable in cases of CSF leakage.
- The wound is closed in layers with muscle and deep fascia in one layer using absorbable sutures (PDS or Vicryl 1 or 0) (Fig. 30.9a).
- Superficial fascia in another layer with Vicryl 2/0 and subcuticular closure of skin (Fig. 30.9b), transverse Steri-Strips and a waterproof dressing are then applied.

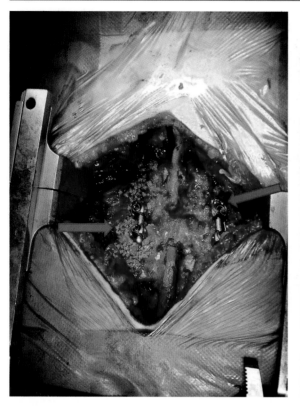 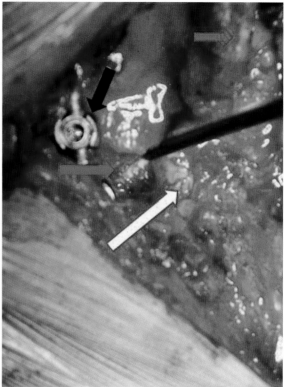

Fig. 30.7 The final decompressed dural sac. The pedicles screws are inserted and longitudinal rods inserted bilaterally. *Blue arrow* illustrates the implanted posterolateral intertransverse bone graft. *Green arrow* illustrates the inserted pedicle screws on the right side

Fig. 30.8 Decompression of the lateral recess at the left L5/S1 region. *Blue arrow* illustrates the middle line (spinous process). *Black arrow* illustrates pedicle screw in situ. *Green arrow* illustrates the exposed left L5 nerve root. *White arrow* illustrates the dural sac

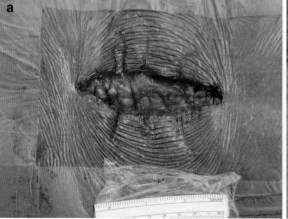 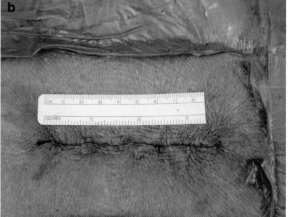

Fig. 30.9 (a) The wound is closed in layers with muscle and deep fascia in one layer using absorbable sutures (PDS or Vicryl 1 or 0). (b) Subcuticular closure of skin

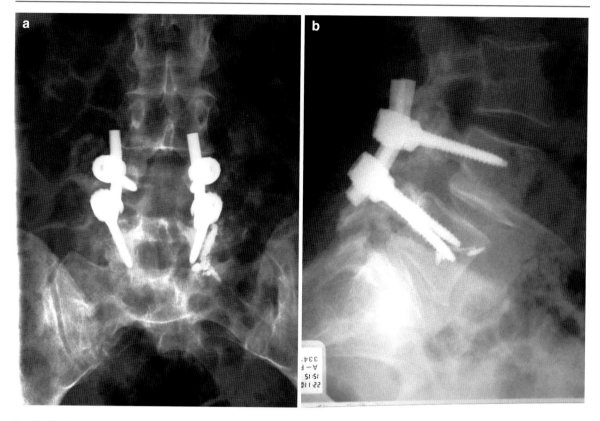

Fig. 30.10 Postoperative X-rays (**a** *AP* and **b** *lateral*) showing the decompressed spine, the spinal instrumentation, and the posterolateral bone graft

Postoperative Care

- After wound dressing, the patient is carefully moved to the trolley into a supine position.
- The anesthesia is reversed and the drain opened.
- Neurological observations and cauda equina observations are performed:
  Every 15 mins for 2 h
  Every 30 mins for 2 h
  Every hour for 2 h
- If all is well at this stage, these observations are performed 4 hourly thereafter.

Rehabilitation

- Patients are usually mobilized on the first postoperative day by the physiotherapists.

- Check radiographs and blood tests are done and the drain removed at 24–48 h depending on drainage (Fig. 30.10a, b).
- When the patient is freely mobile and is voiding normally they are discharged.
- The wound should be kept dry for 12 days.
- Outpatient physiotherapy is used depending on the individual need of the patient.

Outpatient Follow-up

- Patients are routinely reviewed 6 weeks and 12 weeks after surgery.
- If instrumented fusion is performed, follow-up should continue until radiological evidence of bone graft fusion is achieved with 3, 6, and 12 months appointments.

Further Reading

Soegaard R, Bünger CE, Christiansen T, et al. Circumferential fusion is dominant over posterolateral fusion in a long-term perspective: cost-utility evaluation of a randomized controlled trial in severe, chronic low back pain. Spine (Phila Pa 1976). 2007;32(22):2405–14.

Han X, Zhu Y, Cui C, et al. A meta-analysis of circumferential fusion versus instrumented posterolateral fusion in the lumbar spine. Spine (Phila Pa 1976). 2009;34(17):E618–25.

Peng CW, Yue WM, Poh SY, et al. Clinical and radiological outcomes of minimally invasive versus open transforaminal lumbar interbody fusion. Spine (Phila Pa 1976). 2009;34(13):1385–9.

DiPaola CP, Molinari RW. Posterior lumbar interbody fusion. J Am Acad Orthop Surg. 2008;16(3):130–9.

Ozgur BM, Aryan HE, Pimenta L, et al. Extreme Lateral Interbody Fusion (XLIF): a novel surgical technique for anterior lumbar interbody fusion. Spine J. 2006;6(4): 435–43.

Spinal Stenosis/Decompression

31

Efthimios J. Karadimas and Abhay S. Rao

Indications

- Spinal stenosis.
- Disc prolapse with no relative spinal instability.
- Caudal equina syndrome.

Preoperative Planning

Clinical Assessment

- Signs consistent with bilateral lower leg neurological claudication.
- Limited walking capacity – becomes more evident with progressive deterioration of spinal stenosis.
- A detailed neurological examination (sensory level, muscle tone and power, reflexes, bladder and bowel function) is essential to identify the level of disc prolapsed.
- Be alert to identify symptoms consistent with caudal equina (emergency treatment).

Radiological Assessment

- Plain radiographs (AP-Lateral) can provide useful information regarding the level and the degree of degeneration (stenosis).

E.J. Karadimas (✉)
Department of Trauma and Orthopaedic Surgery,
Leeds Teaching Hospitals NHS Trust, Leeds, UK
e-mail: eikaradimas@yahoo.gr

A.S. Rao
Department of Spinal Surgery,
Leeds Teaching Hospitals NHS Trust, Leeds, UK
e-mail: abhay.rao@leedsth.nhs.uk

- Assessment of possible sacralization of the L5 or lumbarization of the S1 vertebra is essential.
- MRI is the diagnostic modality of choice allowing accurate assessment of the level, location (lateral or central), and site of the stenosis, as well as the shape and volume of any protruding disc(s). Visualization of facet joint orientation and hypertrophy can be helpful (Fig. 31.1). Exclusion of pathological causes can also be achieved.

Operative Treatment

Anesthesia

- Patients are operated on under general anesthesia.

Table/Equipment

- Radiolucent table using the "Wilson frame."
- Image intensifier.
- General orthopedic instruments, Kerisson forceps, Cobbs, nerve root retractors, nibblers, curettes, and osteotomes should all be available (Fig. 31.2).
- Head light, loops.
- Epidural patches, durasheal, local hemostatic agents (Surgicel, flosheal, Spongostan).
- A bipolar diathermy must be used for patients with pacemakers.
- Calf pumps are always applied for intraoperative DVT prophylaxis.

P.V. Giannoudis (ed.), *Practical Procedures in Elective Orthopaedic Surgery*,
DOI 10.1007/978-0-85729-820-1_31, © Springer-Verlag London Limited 2012

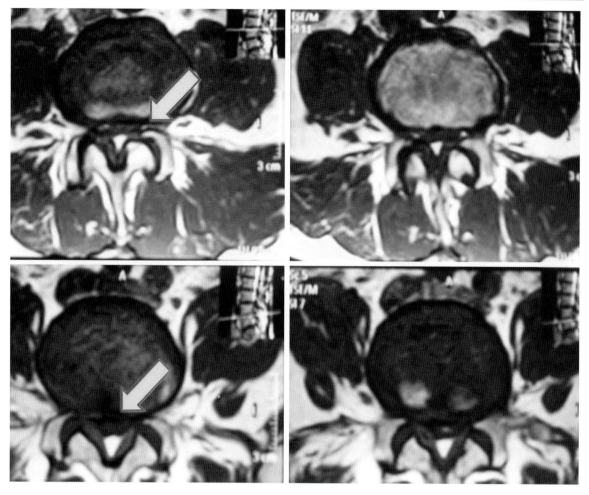

Fig. 31.1 MRI evaluation of the stenotic levels

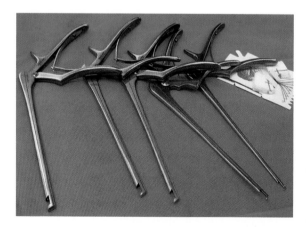

Fig. 31.2 Different sizes of Kerisson forceps

Patient Positioning

- The anesthetist guides the transfer of the patient onto the operating table.
- Caution should be given during the positioning of the patient on the Wilson frame to avoid pressure problems on skin of chest, flanks, and knees (Fig. 31.3).
- Be aware of brachial plexus stretching and pressure on eyes.
- Ensure no pressure applied to abdomen and its contents. This will minimize back pressure from abdominal veins anastomosing with epidural veins.
- Another option is the "kneeling" position, with the advantage of having the posterior lumbar spine elements in distraction, which allows easier access to the stenotic levels and makes the decompression easier (Fig. 31.4).

Fig. 31.3 OSI table with the Wilson frame

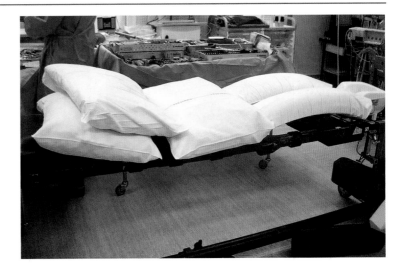

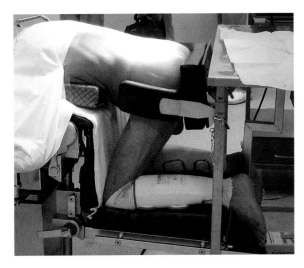

Fig. 31.4 Another option is the "kneeling" position, with the advantage of having the posterior lumbar spine elements in distraction, which allows easier access to the stenotic levels and makes the decompression easier

- The lumbar spine must be parallel to the floor to make the access to the level which is going to be decompressed easier.

Draping

- The skin is cleaned with the use of antiseptic solutions (alcoholic povidone/iodine) from the chest level down to the buttock as well as both sides of the lumbar spine approx. 10–15 cm from the midline (Fig. 31.5).

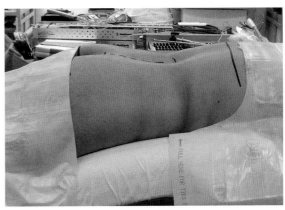

Fig. 31.5 Marking of spinous processes and the length of the incision

Level Checking

- Fluoroscopy must validate the level of the decompression prior to initiation of the procedure.
- Use the image intensifier to check that the operative level is correct.
- Palpate and mark the spinous processes using a marking pen.
- An epidural needle is pushed through the skin perpendicular to the skin surface until near the spinal column. Obtain X-ray image to check position.
- Once the correct disc level is identified, this level is marked with two skin marks perpendicular to the long axis of the spinal column at the level of the disc.

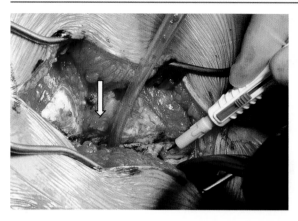

Fig. 31.6 Soft tissue dissection with the use of a cutting diathermy

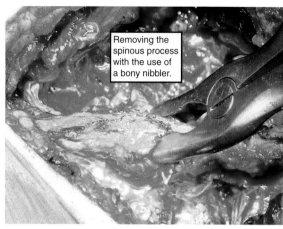

Fig. 31.7 The spinous process is removed using of a bone nibbler

Surgical Exposure

- Perform a straight skin incision over the marked level.
- Divide inner fascia from the spinous processes using either an inside knife or cutting diathermy.
- Using the Cobb retractor and cutting diathermy, detach the erector spinae muscles from the spinous processes (Fig. 31.6) above and below the disc level that is being operated upon and from the interspinous ligament between these spinous processes.
- Extend the dissection to the facet joints.
- Depending on the extension of the decompression, the fascia is divided bilaterally, and in cases of wide decompression, the spinous process of the specific level is removed (Fig. 31.7).
- Swabs compressed with Cobb retractors can be used to tamponate the bleeding and to push the muscles sideways.
- A dip retractor is applied at this stage to facilitate the exposure of the vertebral posterior elements (vertebral laminae).
- Prior to initiation of decompression, it is good practice to re-verify the level of decompression using fluoroscopy.
- Using a Kerrison dissector (no. 2) decompression can be initialized safely from the attachment of the flavum at the lower edge of the proximal vertebral laminae (for L4 decompression – the starting point is the inferior part of L4 lamina).
- Excision of bone is facilitated using bone nibblers.

- Further excision of flavum and bone until exposure of the dural sac is achieved using Kerrison no. 4,5 dissectors.
- Be aware that in cases of severe spinal stenosis there is an increased risk of dura tear.
- As the decompression progresses laterally, avoid damaging the facet joints (Fig. 31.8).
- Note that one-third of the descending facet can be resected bilaterally without destabilizing the spinal column.
- In case that a limited decompression is planned, excision of the lower half of the laminae is recommended.
- If discectomy is indicated, using a nerve retractor, the dural sac is retracted for better exposure of the disc space.
- Using a blade, divide the posterior annulus, and the disc/nuclear material is removed using a pituitary forceps or disc forceps (curved or straight).
- In cases of dural tears, either nonabsorbable sutures 6/0 or dural clips can be used. Alternatively, dura seal can be applied (usually in small tears).
- Usage of drain is common practice, but in cases of dural tear, a nonsuction drain is recommended.

Implant Positioning

- Instrumentation is advisable if the decompression is extensive and includes more than two levels.

Fig. 31.8 Bilateral decompression: *a* dura, *b* spinous process of the adjacent levels

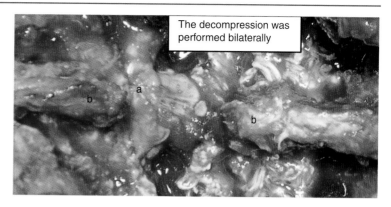

The decompression was performed bilaterally

Closure

- Prior to closure, an epidural catheter could be applied for postoperative pain management.
- A Valsalva test can be used to check that there is no CSF leak or to confirm that a dural tear has sealed.
- Use Vicryl 1 interrupted sutures for the inner layer.
- Continuous or interrupted sutures PDS or Vicryl 2/0 can be used to close the subcutaneous tissues.
- Use 3/0 Monocryl absorbable sutures for the skin.
- Local anesthetic agent (Marcain 0.5%) can be infiltrated around the skin incision for pain relief.

Postoperative Management

- On return to the ward, patients are allowed to mobilize as pain allows.
- Neurological observations and cauda equina observations are performed:
  - Every 15 min for 2 h
  - Every 30 min for 2 h
  - Every hour for 2 h
- Subsequently, assuming that there is no neurological sequelae, these observations are performed 4 hourly thereafter.

- Provided there are no postoperative complications, discharge patient when he has been mobilized satisfactorily by the physiotherapy team.
- Bending and lifting is usually avoided for 6 weeks.

Outpatient Follow-up

- Patients are routinely reviewed 6 weeks after surgery, 3 months, 6 months, and thereafter as indicated per local unit protocol.

Further Reading

Armin SS, Holly LT, Khoo LT. Minimally invasive decompression for lumbar stenosis and disc herniation. Neurosurg Focus. 2008;25(2):E11.

Atlas SJ, Delitto A. Spinal stenosis: surgical versus nonsurgical treatment. Clin Orthop Relat Res. 2006;443:198–207.

Babb A, Carlson WO. Spinal stenosis. S D Med. 2006;59(3):103–5.

Chou R, Baisden J, Carragee EJ, et al. Surgery for low back pain: a review of the evidence for an American Pain Society Clinical Practice Guideline. Spine (Phila Pa 1976). 2009;34(10):1094–109.

Siddiqui M, Karadimas E, Nicol M, et al. Influence of X Stop on neural foramina and spinal canal area in spinal stenosis. Spine (Phila Pa 1976). 2006;31(25):2958–62.

Part VI

Spine: Scoliosis

Posterior Correction of Adolescent Idiopathic Scoliosis (Principles for the Posterior Correction of Spinal Curvatures)

Robert A. Dunsmuir

Introduction

- Correction of scoliosis deformities can be performed by anterior or posterior approaches.
- This chapter describes the posterior approach, which is the commonest approach to the spine for this type of surgery.
- The decision about the need for anterior surgery or anterior surgery combined with posterior surgery is beyond the scope of this book.
- This chapter describes the salient features common to all posterior corrective procedures.
- Surgery for neuromuscular scoliosis or congenital scoliosis is not considered in this chapter.

Indications

- Adolescent idiopathic scoliosis.
- Thoracic scoliosis – single or double curves.
- Thoracolumbar scoliosis.
- Double structural scoliosis (Fig. 32.1).
- Lumbar scoliosis.

R.A. Dunsmuir
Department of Trauma and Orthopaedic Surgery,
Leeds Teaching Hospitals NHS Trust,
Leeds, UK
e-mail: robert.dunsmuir@leedsth.nhs.uk

Preoperative Planning

Clinical Assessment

- The patient will present with a scoliotic deformity requesting correction.
- Generally, these deformities are painless; therefore if pain is part of the presenting complaint, then other potential pain sources should be sought.
- In idiopathic scoliosis, there is no compression of the spinal cord or spinal nerve.
- Neurological symptoms, such as paresthesia, muscle weakness, or bladder/bowel dysfunction, should alert the treating surgeon to other causes for this neurological dysfunction.
- In girls, ask if menstruation has begun. If so, this suggests that the curve is less likely to progress.
  On examination, the surgeon should look for
  1. Is the spine balanced? If *balanced*, the occipital protuberance will sit directly vertically above the natal cleft. If it is not, the spine is *unbalanced*.
  2. The rib hump is generally on the right side of the posterior chest wall. A loin hump is generally on the left side of the posterior abdominal wall. In some cases, the opposite may apply to both deformities.
  3. Determine if the shoulders are level. If the patient has a right thoracic curve, their right shoulder is generally elevated above the left shoulder. In the presence of a right thoracic curve, if the left shoulder is elevated above the right or the shoulders are level, it would suggest the presence of a higher thoracic curve above the main curve.
  4. Look for signs of underlying spinal dysraphism (hairy patches, sinus, nevi, etc.) or signs of other

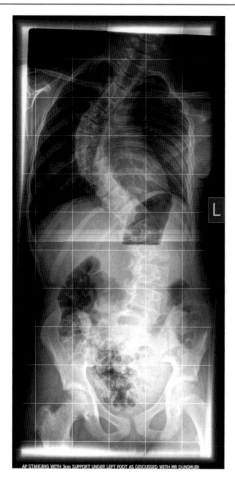

AP STANDING WITH 3cm SUPPORT UNDER LEFT FOOT AS DISCUSSED WITH MR DUNSMUIR

Fig. 32.1 AP X-ray of a double structural scoliosis

neurological conditions (café au lait spots >5, axillary freckling).
5. Look for signs of secondary sexual characteristics.
6. Bend the spine from side to side to assess the flexibility of the curve.
7. Perform a forward bending test to assess the rib hump.

Radiological Assessment

- Obtain X-rays of the whole spine AP and lateral, with the patient standing. These films will show the whole spine and all the scoliotic curves.
- The stiffness of the curves is determined by obtaining X-rays of the thoracic and lumbar spine, with the patient bent maximally in the coronal plane to the right and the left.
- Using these bending films, the upper and lower limits of the area of the spine to be instrumented can be determined.

- Preoperatively, an MRI scan of the whole spine is obtained. This scan is used to look for the presence of spinal anomalies – Arnold–Chiari malformation, syrinx, diastematomyelia and tethered cord. Any of these abnormalities may increase the risk of neurological damage during surgery or prevent surgery from occurring.

Classification

- Numerous classification systems have been developed to assess idiopathic scoliosis.
- Scoliosis is usually divided into *Infantile* (birth–3 years), *Juvenile* (3–10 years), or *Adolescent* (>10 years) by the age at which the condition is first diagnosed. Some surgeons classify idiopathic scoliosis into *Early onset* (<10 years old) and *Late onset* (10 years or older) again by age at diagnosis.
- The curves can be classified by the anatomical position of the apex of the curve (the most laterally displaced vertebra in the curve):
   Thoracic scoliosis – single or double curves
   Thoracolumbar scoliosis
   Double structural scoliosis
   Lumbar scoliosis
- The curve patterns can be classified using published classification systems. The King classification system has been used for many years. This has been largely superceded by the Lenke classification system.

Choosing Fusion Levels

- The level of arthrodesis usually extends from the neutral vertebra at the top of the curve to the neutral vertebra at the bottom of the curve. In addition to this, the lowest limit of the arthrodesis must stop at a vertebra that transects a line drawn vertically upward from the center of the sacrum – the center sacral line (Fig. 32.2).

Operative Treatment

Anesthesia

- Patients are operated under general anesthesia.
- As the patient will be "prone" throughout the procedure, it is necessary to use endotracheal intubation with an *armored* endotracheal tube.

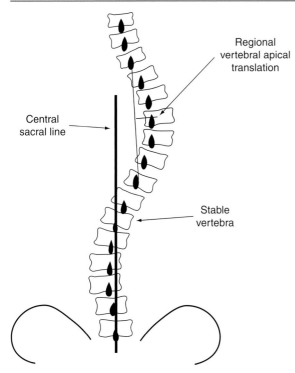

Central sacral line

Regional vertebral apical translation

Stable vertebra

Fig. 32.2 The center sacral line. The *perpendicular line* to the proximal sacrum transects the L3 vertebra. The inferior limit of the arthrodesis should come to this level

- A CVP line and an arterial line are required for close intraoperative monitoring by the anesthetist.
- The patient is usually catheterized to monitor urine output.
- During the operation, a "Cell Saver" is used to minimize the amount of allograft blood used intraoperatively.

Spinal Cord Monitoring (Fig. 32.3)

- Intraoperative spinal cord monitoring is used throughout the operation.
- Somatosensory evoked potentials are used as standard in most countries (motor evoked potentials are commonly used in the United States and will become standard as the technology becomes more available). The electrodes are glued to the scalp and ankles. This allows constant real-time monitoring of the sensory tracts in the spinal cord. It allows early detection of abnormalities in function of the spinal cord during the operation. These are most likely to occur during

the deformity correction procedure and the placement of spinal implants.

Patient Positioning

- The preferred choice is a "Jackson table" (Fig. 32.4). This allows adequate image intensifier visualization of the upper thoracic vertebrae for placement of pedicles screws, if these are required.
- The choice of operating table is largely determined by the instrumentation to be used. If pedicle, laminar, and transverse process hooks are to be used in the upper thoracic spine, then a Wilson frame can be used as this will allow radiological visualization of the vertebrae from the lower thoracic spine distally.
- The anesthetist guides and leads the transfer of the patient onto the operating table. The patient is rolled prone onto the operating table on top of the supporting cushions. The patient's head is rested in the ProneView.
- Pneumatic calf pumps are always applied for intraoperative DVT prophylaxis.

Precautions

- Ensure there is no pressure on the patient's axillae.
- Ensure that the patient's knees and ankles are not overextended.
- Ensure the patient's eyes are visible using the"ProneView". The patient can "slip" distally during this procedure, and pressure can be applied to the orbits.
- Ensure no pressure is applied to abdomen and its contents. This will minimize back pressure from abdominal veins anastomosing with epidural veins.
- Ensure there is no traction on the upper limbs and the brachial plexus.

Potential Problems

Pressure problems on skin of chest, flanks, anterior superior iliac spines, and knees

Brachial plexus stretching

Pressure on eyes

Fig. 32.3 The display on the monitor of the SSEP cord monitoring is illustrated

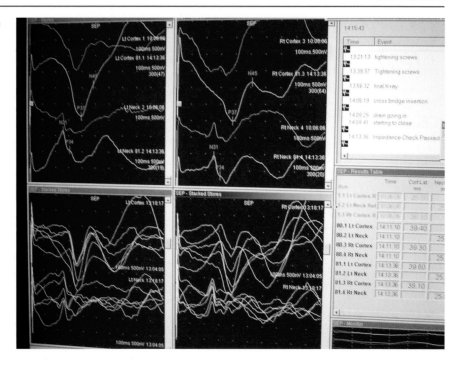

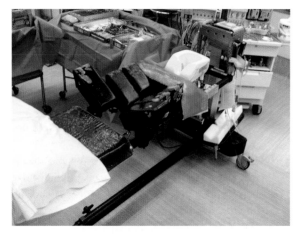

Fig. 32.4 The Jackson table is shown. This illustration demonstrates the "ProneView" to support the head. There are a superior chest support and a number of wedges to support the remainder of the chest, abdomen, and pelvis

Instrumentation

- Numerous spinal instrumentation systems are available. The choice of system is determined by the surgeon's training and experience.

Skin Marking

- An indelible marker is used to show the tips of the spinous processes. A curvilinear "incision" is marked with an indelible skin marker to show the incision to be made. The incision is made at the midline but must be gently curved to accommodate the scoliotic curve(s) (Fig. 32.5).

Draping

- The skin is prepped with the antiseptic solution of choice.
- Adhesive paper drapes are applied, and the operative field covered with an occlusive dressing (e.g., Opsite) (Fig. 32.6).

Surgical Exposure

- The skin is incised along the preselected line. Epidermis and dermis are incised until the thoracolumbar fascia is identified. All the spinous processes are exposed along the complete length of the wound.

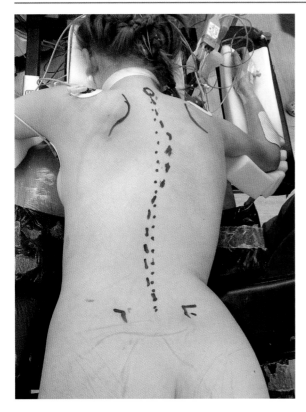

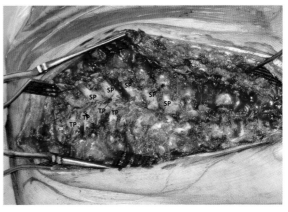

Fig. 32.7 The erector spinae dissected from the spine to expose all transverse processes over the selected fusion area

Fig. 32.5 The skin marks (*dashes* are made to show the spinous processes and to highlight to scoliotic curves). The incision site is marked as a curvilinear incision (*dots*)

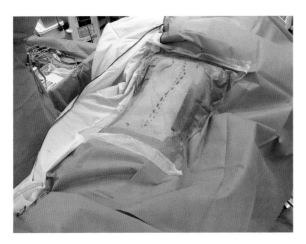

Fig. 32.6 The operating field fully draped

- The cartilaginous apophysis on the tip of each spinous process is divided longitudinally using sharp dissection. The soft tissue between these incisions is divided by monopolar diathermy.

- Starting distally, each cartilaginous cap is peeled from the bony spinous process using a Cobb resector. This allows the periosteum on the spinous process to be peeled from the bone. This process of peeling the periosteum from bone can be extended along the lamina toward the facet joint. The adjacent spinous process is similarly treated. The remaining soft tissue between adjacent spinous processes can be detached by monopolar diathermy or blunt dissection using Lexel biters.

- The above process is repeated at each level up the spine on both sides.

- The vertebrae should be exposed to show the transverse processes over those levels of the spine to be arthrodesed (Fig. 32.7).

- All facet joints are excised, and transverse process-es are detached from the vertebrae and their rib attachments. This action increases the flexibility of the spine.

- The spine is then instrumented at the chosen levels. The instrumentation used is determined by each surgeon. Laminar hooks (supralaminar or infralaminar), transverse process hooks, pedicle hooks, and pedicle screws can all be used to correct a scoliotic deformity. A combination of these anchorage points is commonly used depending on surgeon's experience, the flexibility of the spine, and the size of pedicles.

- Pedicle screws are inserted using the image intensifier to help guide safe screw placement (Fig. 32.8). Experienced surgeons may insert screws without the help of an image intensifier. The entry point for

Fig. 32.8 Using the image intensifier to help placement on pedicle screws

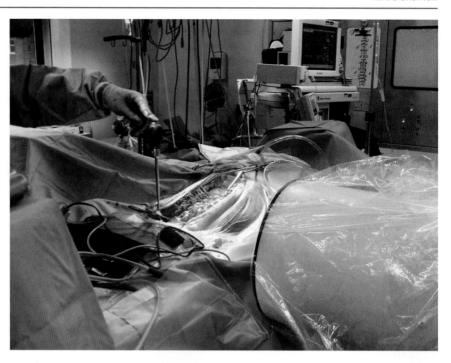

pedicle screws is determined by the vertebra being instrumented.

- We will tend to use construct devised entirely of pedicle screws unless the pedicle is too narrow to accept a screw. In these cases, we will use a pedicle or laminar hook (Fig. 32.9a).
- Once all the anchorage points are secured, two rods (*one for each* side of the spine) are contoured to a shape approximating to a normal sagittal profile. These rods are secured to the pedicle screws and laminar/pedicle hooks but still allowing rotation within the head of the screw/hook.
- The long rods are rotated to straighten the spine. Once happy with the correction, the rods are secured in place with locking nuts (Fig. 32.9b).
- The spinous processes are excised, and the dorsal surfaces of the laminae are decorticated. The bone obtained from this action can be used as autograft. The autograft can be mixed with an artificial bone substitute. The resulting mixture is then placed over the decorticated laminae from the top to the bottom of the instrumented area. Cross-link connectors are placed proximally and distally to both rods (Fig. 32.9c).

Closure

- Two drains are inserted into the wound. The wound is closed in layers – thoracolumbar fascia, subcutaneous tissues, and skin.
- Since this operation is largely about cosmesis, a subcuticular suture for skin closure is the preferred method of closure.
- The final clinical result is visible at the end of the procedure (Fig. 32.10a, b).
- Wound is kept dry for the first 12 postoperative days.

Postoperative Observations

- Neurological observations and cauda equina observations are performed:
  Every 15 min for 2 h
  Every 30 min for 2 h
  Every hour for 2 h
- If all is well at this stage these observations are performed 4 hourly thereafter.
- On return to the ward, patients are allowed to mobilize as pain permits. Routine postoperative blood

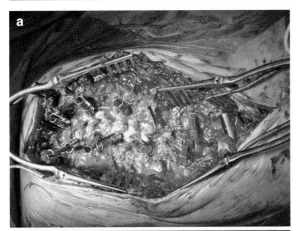

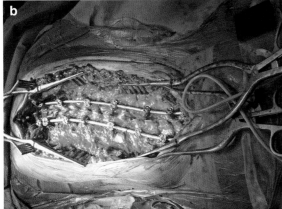

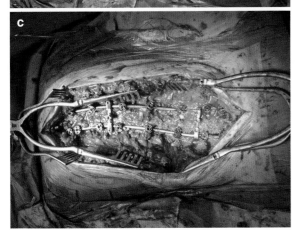

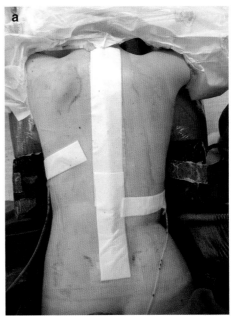

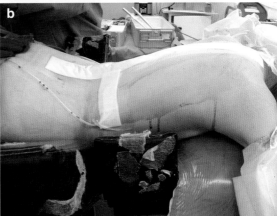

Fig. 32.10 (a) Posterior view of correction achieved at the end of operation. (b) Lateral view of correction achieved

tests (U&Es, FBC, coagulation) are performed until the patient is eating and drinking well.

Rehabilitation

- When the patient is freely mobile and is voiding normally they are discharged. Before discharge, a standing X-ray of the whole spine is obtained (Fig. 32.11).

Fig. 32.9 (a) Pedicle screws inserted into chosen anchorage points. (b) The final construct and correction before bone grafting, and (c) Final construct with screws, rods, bone graft, and cross links in situ. The spinous processes have been excised and the laminae decorticated. The autograft bone has been mixed with a bone substitute and placed over the decorticated bones

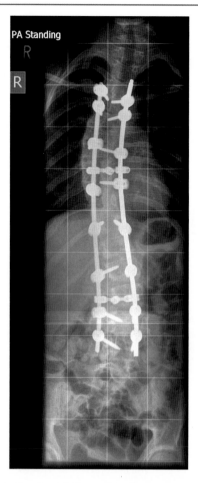

Fig. 32.11 Standing AP X-ray of the final correction

Outpatient Follow-up

- Patients are routinely reviewed 6 weeks after surgery.
- Further review occurs at 3 months, 6 months, and 1 year postoperatively.
- X-rays are taken at the second and fourth postoperative visits to determine progress of spinal fusion.
- Follow-up is required until there is X-ray evidence of a solid fusion over the instrumented area of the spine.

Further Reading

Nachemson A. A long term follow-up study of non-treated scoliosis. Acta Orthop Scand. 1968;39:466–76.

King HA, Moe JH, Bradford DS. The selection of fusion levels in thoracic idiopathic scoliosis. JBJS Am. 1983;65:1302–10.

Lenke LG, Betz RR, Harms J, Bridwell KH, Clements DH, Lowe TG, et al. Adolescent Idiopathic Scoliosis: a new classification system to determine the extent of spinal arthrodesis. JBJS Am. 2001;83:1169–81.

Aebi M, Thalgott JS, Webb JK. AO ASIF principles in spinal surgery. New York, Berlin: AO Publishing, Springer; 1998. p. 58, 102–105.

Surgical Technique of Vertebral Cement Augmentation (Vertebro/Kyphoplasty)

33

Antony L. R. Michael, Abhay S. Rao, and Jake Timothy

Introduction

- The debilitating nature of pain after vertebral compression fracture both due to osteoporosis and metastatic disease is well documented in the literature.
- Vertebroplasty and kyphoplasty are two techniques for augmenting of vertebral bodies with acrylic bone cement.
- The aim of the procedure is to stabilize the vertebral fracture and thus relieve pain.
- A biopsy may be carried out at the time of cement augmentation.
- It is generally done as a day case procedure.

Indications

- Osteoporotic vertebral compression fractures where early pain relief is desirable.

A.L.R. Michael (✉)
Department of Trauma and Orthopaedics,
Leeds Teaching Hospitals NHS Trust,
Leeds, UK
e-mail: arexmichael@yahoo.co.uk

A.S. Rao
Department of Spinal Surgery,
Leeds Teaching Hospitals NHS Trust,
Leeds, UK
e-mail: abhay.rao@leedsth.nhs.uk

J. Timothy
Department of Neurosurgery,
Leeds Teaching Hospitals NHS Trust,
Leeds, UK

- Metastatic vertebral fractures that have collapsed or are at imminent danger of collapse.
- Augmentation of pedicle screws in severe osteoporosis.

Relative Contraindications

- Fractures with deficient posterior wall and fractures/vertebral lesions that have defects that will not contain the cement.
- Infection in the spine.
- Vertebra plana.

Preoperative Assessment

History

- Record history of the presenting complaint, comorbidities, and requirement of pain relief.
- The nature, site, and radiation of pain should be carefully ascertained.
- The duration of symptoms is important as recent evidence suggests that intervention is not significantly effective in longstanding conditions.
- It is advisable to obtain objective scoring systems at this stage to permit postoperative assessment of outcome.

Clinical Examination

- Follow the time honored sequence of look, feel, and move.
- Assess neurological status and be aware that pain may be referred distally.

P.V. Giannoudis (ed.), *Practical Procedures in Elective Orthopaedic Surgery*,
DOI 10.1007/978-0-85729-820-1_33, © Springer-Verlag London Limited 2012

Fig. 33.1 The marking and preparation of the patient is shown. The patient is positioned prone. The level to be treated is marked with fluoroscopy, and this area is prepared with a suitable solution. Alcoholic iodine solutions are used at our institution; the area is draped

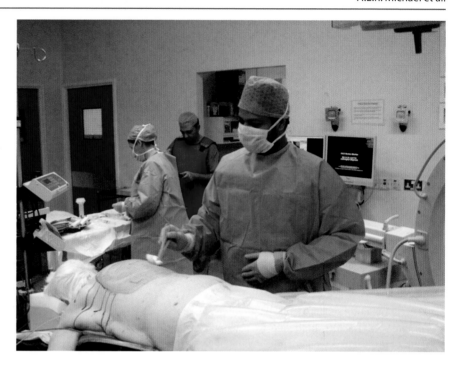

- There is usually localized tenderness at the level of the lesion.
- Routine blood tests, inflammatory markers, bone profile, and coagulation studies are useful.

Radiological Investigations

- MRI can determine the nature of the fracture and the effect on the neural elements (Short Tau Inversion Recovery (STIR) sequence is believed to be indicative of recent/symptomatic vertebral fracture especially when there are multiple compression fractures of doubtful chronology and symptomatology).
- CT gives better definition of bony involvement especially if the integrity of the posterior vertebral wall is in question.
- Isotope bone scan is very sensitive but nonspecific.
- Postprocedural CT, venography, and investigations for cement embolization are not routinely required.

Surgical Technique

Anesthesia

- The procedure is carried out in the operating theater or angiogram suite.
- Sedation or light general anesthesia is preferable.

- It is supplemented by local anesthesia at sites of skin puncture.

Position

- Patient is placed prone on a radiolucent table, with a patient support frame (Fig. 33.1).
- There should be space for the C-arm fluoroscopy to swing from anteroposterior (AP) to lateral.
- Biplanar fluoroscopy is useful but may restrict access for the surgeon.
- It is important that high quality fluoroscopy is available and the operator is familiar with the requirements of the procedure.

Preparation

- Sterile preparation and draping are carried out. Check with the C-arm that true AP and lateral images can be obtained (Fig. 33.2a, b).
- The vertebral body should be visualized with the two pedicles and the spinous process seen as the eyes and beak of an owl.
- The vertebroplasty or kyphoplasty kit of choice and all instruments and cement required should be available.
- The scrub nurse should be familiar with the kit and the procedure.

Fig. 33.2 (**a**, **b**) Infiltration of local anesthetic at sites of skin puncture located under fluoroscopy. The skin puncture site is chosen lateral to the pedicles so that when the converging needles reach the entry point for the pedicles they will be at the upper lateral quadrant of the pedicle as seen on AP fluoroscopy (10 o'clock and 2 o'clock for left and right, respectively)

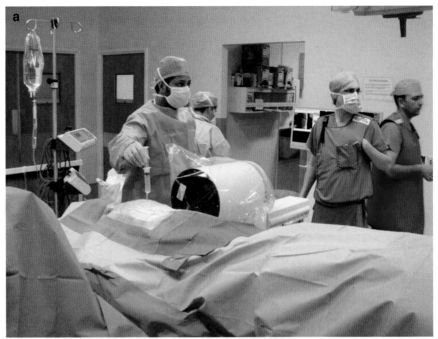

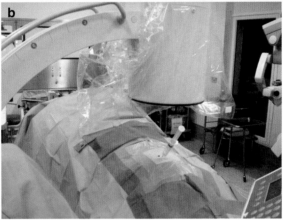

Access

- The trocar that has been selected may be introduced through one pedicle (unipedicular) for vertebroplasty and through two pedicles (bipedicular) for kyphoplasty (Fig. 33.3a, b).
- If the pedicle appearance is likened to a clockface, the trocar is introduced in the 10 o'clock position on the left and 2 o'clock position on the right side.
- It is introduced with a medial angulation so as not to breach the medial wall but to end up close to the midline in the vertebral body.
- All advancement of the trocar should be monitored by orthogonal fluoroscopy (Fig. 33.4a, b).

- Once the trocar is in a satisfactory position, the preparation for cement injection is carried out depending on whether it is a vertebroplasty or a kyphoplasty procedure.
- In vertebroplasty, the inner needle is removed leaving the outer sheath of the trocar in place.
- The cement is then mixed and introduced via the introducer when it has reached the correct consistency for injection, usually of a toothpaste consistency.
- This varies between the different types of kit used; hence, it is recommended that the manufacturer's guidelines are followed.
- The introduction of cement should be done slowly and deliberately under fluoroscopy guidance

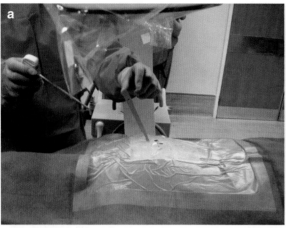 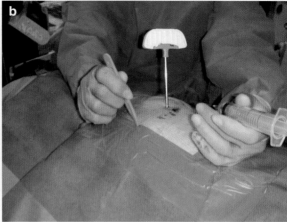

Fig. 33.3 (**a**, **b**) Shows skin incision followed by trocar insertion. The skin incision is placed at the selected site and is approximately 5 mm long to allow the trocar to be passed. The trocar is advanced until bone is felt and fluoroscopy used to verify the correct approach to the pedicle. In vertebroplasty, one trocar is used and aimed to reach as close to the midline of the vertebral body as possible. In kyphoplasty, bipedicular approach with two trocars is carried out

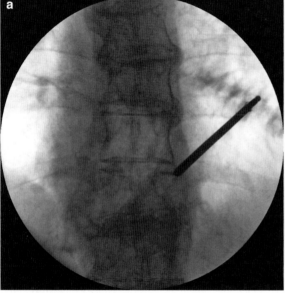 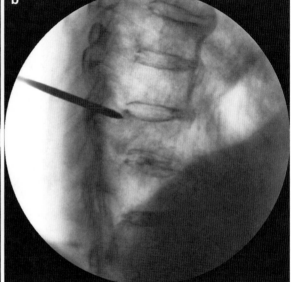

Fig. 33.4 (**a**, **b**) Insertion of trocar and orthogonal images. Once the trocar strikes bone, orthogonal imaging is required to ensure that they follow the optimum path. On AP the medial wall of the pedicle should only be crossed when the tip of the trocar is seen to go past the pedicle and into the vertebral body on lateral views. If the medial wall is breached before this, it means that the medial wall of the pedicle has been breached and there is risk of neurological injury

keeping a careful lookout for any cement leakage through the vertebrobasilar veins.
- If there were any defects identified in the vertebral wall, these should be observed carefully, and injection stopped if there is any risk of extravasation.
- Injection is stopped when there has been adequate filling of the vertebral body.

- Approximately 3 mL of cement is adequate for augmenting one vertebral body.
- The inner needle is placed in the trocar before withdrawal to prevent cement backflow into the pedicles.
- In kyphoplasty a bipedicular access is used.
- Two trocars are introduced into the vertebral body under fluoroscopic guidance (Fig. 33.5a–d).

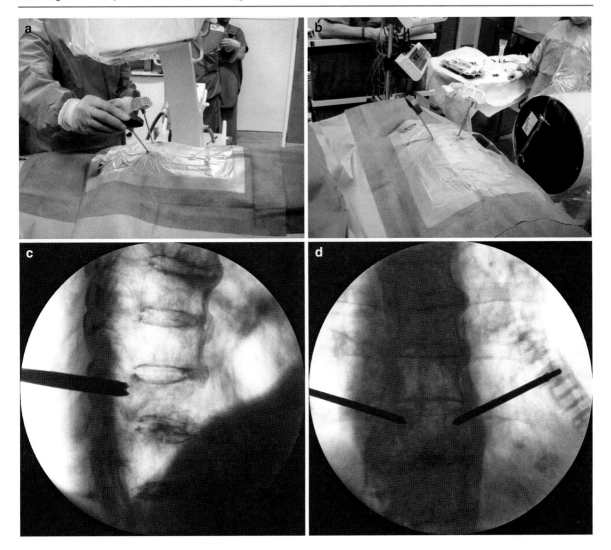

Fig. 33.5 (**a–d**) Insertion of second trocar and confirmation of satisfactory position

- Once optimum position has been reached, the inner needles are removed, and a handheld drill is used to create a path for the balloons (Fig. 33.6a, b).
- A tamp is used to clear any debris from the path. The balloons are then introduced into the prepared path in the vertebral body (Fig. 33.7a–d).
- The balloons are attached to a prefilled syringe with contrast material with a pressure display.
- The balloons are inflated with the contrast under fluoroscopy control to effect some restoration of height and create a cavity for the bone cement (Fig. 33.8a–d).
- There are maximum volumes and pressure recommendations from the manufacturer, and these should be adhered to very strictly to avoid balloon rupture

which will release the contrast into the vertebral body making monitoring of cement injection difficult.
- Once the balloons have been inflated satisfactorily, the cement is mixed and the volume to be injected is read from the syringe with contrast corresponding to the amount of contrast that was used to inflate the balloons (Fig. 33.9a, b).
- The balloons are then sequentially deflated and withdrawn.
- Cement is then injected into the void/cavity created by the balloons under careful fluoroscopic monitoring (Fig. 33.10a, b).
- Once cement injection is complete, the needles are introduced into the trocar to withdraw them without allowing cement to back flow.

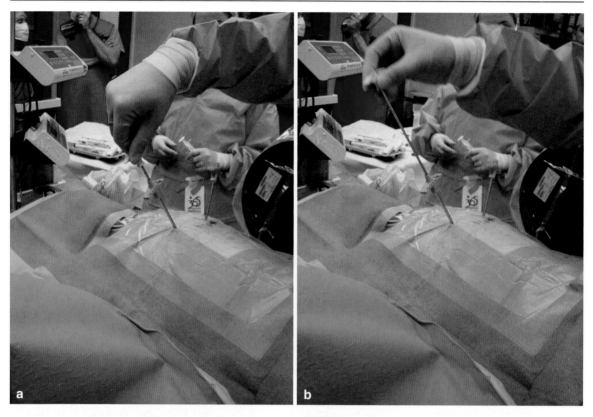

Fig. 33.6 (**a, b**) Drilling and tamping for balloon path. This step is not required for a vertebroplasty. For kyphoplasty, a path needs to be created for the balloons; this is done with a handheld drill which is introduced into the vertebral body past the outer sleeve of the trocar, and hence this part of the procedure should be done with fluoroscopy to avoid breaching the anterior vertebral wall. Once the path is drilled, a tamp is used to clear bone debris from the drill path; this is an important step to reduce the risk of sharp bone fragments tearing the balloons

Postoperative Care

- Patients are monitored in a postoperative observation area with frequent neurological examination.
- They are allowed to mobilize when the effects of sedation/anesthetic have worn off.

Follow-up

- Routine follow-up is done at 6 weeks, 3 months, and 6 months from procedure.

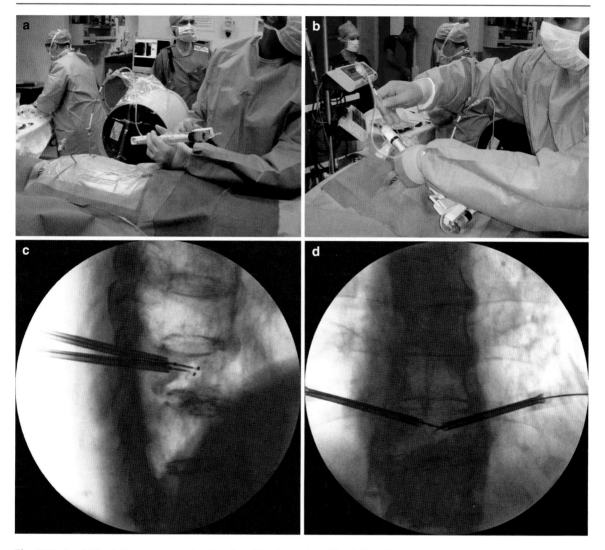

Fig. 33.7 (**a–d**) The balloons are introduced and position is checked. The deflated balloons connected to the contrast syringe are introduced into the path created in the vertebral body; the position is confirmed by fluoroscopy

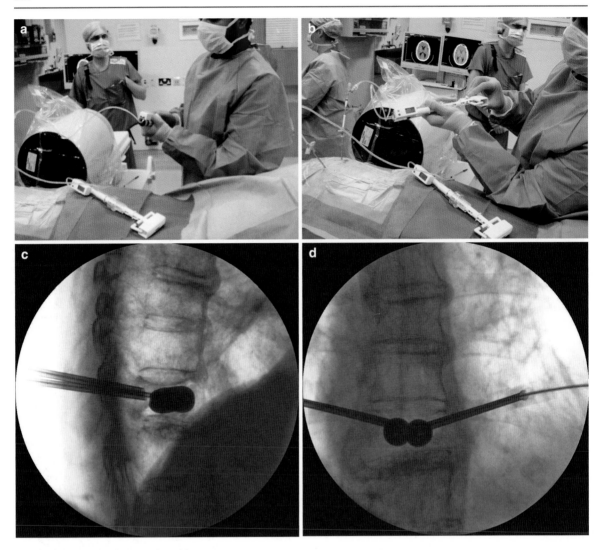

Fig. 33.8 (**a–d**) The balloons are inflated with contrast and the pressure and position checked. The balloons are inflated under fluoroscopic guidance. It is important to inflate slowly and steadily. The syringe is supplied with a pressure monitor; the volume of contrast used can be read from the syringe. Fluoroscopy is used to check that the balloons are sited optimally during inflation. The final volume of contrast used to achieve balloon dilation is noted as this is the volume of cement that will be used

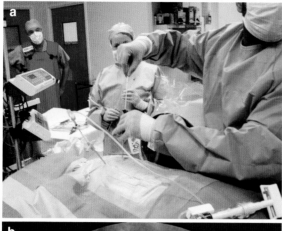

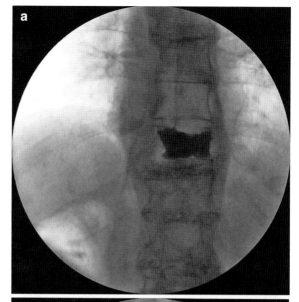

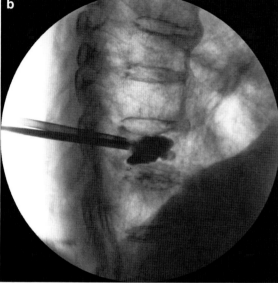

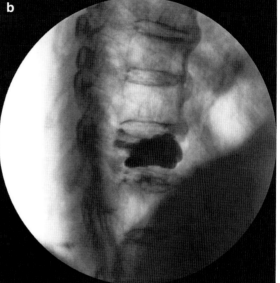

Fig. 33.9 (**a**, **b**) Cement is injected after the balloons have been deflated and removed. When optimum correction of vertebral height is achieved or when the pressure reaches maximum advisable levels, the balloons are sequentially deflated and withdrawn. The cement is supplied in tubes of 1.5 mL, and it is injected under fluoroscopic guidance to ensure that there is no extravertebral leak. Once the predetermined volume of cement is injected, the trocar is withdrawn with the stillette inserted to avoid backflow into the pedicles

Fig. 33.10 (**a**, **b**) Final radiographic result at completion of procedure

Further Reading

Galibert P, Deramond H, Rosat P, LeGars D. Preliminary on the treatment of vertebral angioma by percutaneous acrylic vertebroplasty. Neurochirurgie. 1987;33:166–8.

Phillips FM. Minimally invasive treatments of osteoporotic vertebral compression fractures. Spine. 2003;28(15S):S45–53.

Kallmes DF, Jensen ME. Percutaneous Vertebroplasty, How I Do It. Radiology. 2003;229:27–36.

Index